The Toolbox for Portfolio Development

A practical guide for the primary healthcare team

Roger Pietroni

Foreword by
Sir Donald Irvine
President, General Medical Council

RADCLIFFE MEDICAL PRESS

Radcliffe Medical Press
18 Marcham Road, Abingdon, Oxon OX14 1AA

British Library Cataloguing in Publication Data

A catalogue record for this book is available from the British Library.

ISBN 1 85775 444 1

Typeset by Joshua Associates Ltd, Oxford
Printed and bound by TJ International Ltd, Padstow, Cornwall

Contents

Foreword   vi
About the author   vii
Acknowledgements   viii
List of abbreviations   ix

Introduction   1

Part One: Portfolio-based learning in primary care 5

1 How adults learn best: the importance of reflection   7
2 What is *The Toolbox for Portfolio Development*?   15
3 Identifying learning needs and personal education plans 21
4 What is the role of a 'helper' in keeping a portfolio? 29
5 The primary healthcare team as a learning organisation 33
6 Tips on time management and on keeping a portfolio   37
7 Addressing clinical governance   43

Part Two: Your personal and practice profile   53

Personal profile   55
Practice profile   61

Part Three: The learning activity templates   67

How to use the templates   69

Section A: Learning from patients   71

   For all members of the primary healthcare team
   A1 and A2   Identifying individual strengths and weaknesses
            (self-appraisal for non-clinical topics) and a
            personal education plan   72

A3   Patient interaction logs: identifying needs   78
A4   Significant event analysis   80
A5 and A6   Learning from negatives: complaints, mistakes or
              near misses   83
A7   Learning from positives   86
A8   Learning from audits   87

For clinical members

A9 and A10   Identifying individual strengths and weaknesses
              (self-appraisal for clinical topics) and a personal
              education plan   92
A11 and A12   Consultation analysis: self-assessment   98
A13 and A14   Consultation analysis: patient assessment   102
A15   Learning from PACT data   105

Section B: Learning from colleagues   109

For all members of the primary healthcare team

B1 and B2   Identifying practice strengths and weaknesses and
              a practice education plan   110
B3   Learning from outside events   118
B4   Inter-professional learning   122
B5   In-house education events   124
B6   Learning with other practices   124
B7, B8 and B9 Appraisals   127
B10   Development of guidelines or protocols   143
B11   Learning from external guidelines (National Service
              Frameworks)   146
B12   Learning from risk management   149
B13   Critical reading   152

For clinical members

B14   Critical reading: scientific/clinical articles   156
B15   Consultation analysis: video analysis   161

Section C: Learning from our personal experiences and life events   165

Section D: Addressing clinical governance   167
    Quality assurance   167
    Clinical audit   168
    Clinical effectiveness   169
    Clinical risk management   170
    Staff and organisational development   171

Part Four: Appendices   **173**

Appendix 1   Teacher portfolios   175
Appendix 2   Revalidation for doctors   179
Appendix 3   Useful names, addresses and websites   181

References   189

Index   193

Foreword

Roger Pietroni has written a truly excellent book. *The Toolbox for Portfolio Development* is one of the most important training texts to come out of primary care in recent years, and I am sure it will be widely welcomed by all those working in primary healthcare.

Primary healthcare provides a rich seam of learning experience that can often go untapped. By keeping a portfolio we can record some of this experience and capture it for our own development. A record of this kind enables reflection, and it is through reflection of our own practice that we can best develop good practice.

When primary healthcare teams can learn effectively together, the culture of medicine can be changed for the better. A learning culture that nurtures individual and collective professional development can nourish individual doctors' professionalism. But professional development is no longer our business alone. In today's world we need to show that we are accountable as doctors for the quality of care we provide. In this context records of continuing professional development, as in a portfolio, are critical in demonstrating our continuing fitness to practise.

Given the changing culture of medicine, and the move towards more explicit measures of quality in healthcare, developing individual portfolios is essential. Portfolios will form a key piece of the evidence of continuing fitness to practise required to revalidate in future with the General Medical Council.

Roger Pietroni's book provides a flexible guide to portfolio development, and is not just for doctors but for all those involved in primary healthcare teams. I wish it well and hope that the practical lessons learnt can nourish a new generation of quality-minded primary healthcare teams.

Sir Donald Irvine
October 2000

About the author

Dr Roger Pietroni has been a general practitioner since 1974 and is currently working in a health centre in Ealing, London. He has a wide range of interests within primary care (chronic disease management, psychological medicine) but his principal area of expertise has been in general practice education and training.

In 1992, he obtained a Masters in Medical Education. He has been a GP Trainer, Course Organiser and Associate Adviser (Sub Dean) and is currently working as a Senior Teaching Fellow at Imperial College School of Medicine. As a Member and Fellow of the Royal College of General Practitioners, he has been involved in College affairs and is the author of two RCGP Occasional Papers on Higher Professional Education and Portfolio-based Learning. He has published numerous papers, on educational research (Portfolio-based Learning and Mentoring) and on clinical areas (diabetes and patient education) and is co-editor of *PatientWise* (Wiley, 1995), a compendium of information leaflets for patients. He runs courses on portfolio development from his health centre.

Acknowledgements

Having been involved with portfolios for over 10 years, the most frequent question I have been asked has been 'How does one start a portfolio?' or 'What does a portfolio look like?' It was Norman Mailer who said that writing a book was the closest men got to childbearing. The idea for a book to provide a structure or a toolbox to help individuals develop their own portfolio has had an extraordinarily long gestation period. The fact that it has resulted in a live birth is thanks to a number of people. I am particularly grateful to my wife Jackie, for her encouragement, suggestions and proofreading. I am also grateful to Ealing Park Health Centre, the primary healthcare team and the patients who have been willing guinea pigs in many of the templates and whose refinements have been helpful.

I would like to thank Sir Donald Irvine (revalidation for doctors), Professor John Howie (patient enablement instrument), Dave Boud (hints on keeping a portfolio), Dr Suzanne Kurtz, Dr Jonathan Silverman and Dr Juliet Draper (Calgary–Cambridge guide), Dr Michael Greco (DISQ), Dr Robert Clarke (critical reading guide) and Carla Treloar (teacher portfolios) for their comments and kind permission to use material from their research and work.

List of abbreviations

CHI   Commission for Health Improvement
DISQ   Doctors' interpersonal skills questionnaire
GMC   General Medical Council
HA   health authority
HImP   Health Improvement Programme
NHS   National Health Service
NICE   National Institute for Clinical Excellence
NSF   National Service Frameworks
PACT   Prescribing analysis and cost
PAM   Profession allied to medicine
PCG   Primary care group
PCT   Primary care trust
PEI   Patient enablement instrument
PGEA   Postgraduate Education Allowance
PHCT   Primary healthcare team

Introduction

There is increasing pressure for all people in the health service to begin to develop their own portfolios. Three factors appear to be driving this development.

The first relates to continuing professional development. It is increasingly becoming recognised that keeping a portfolio can not only be a valuable process of learning but will also provide a log and evidence of learning. Nursing and many other professions have been involved in portfolio development for some years, but doctors have been slow to embrace this concept of further learning. The chief medical officer's report on *A Review of Continuing Professional Development in General Practice* (1998)[1] suggests that the Postgraduate Education Allowance (PGEA for doctors) will be removed and replaced by practice and personal education plans or portfolios.

The second factor encouraging the development of portfolios in primary care is clinical governance.[2] Clinical governance involves all health professionals and evidence will need to be produced by primary healthcare teams (PHCTs) to demonstrate that it is being addressed. A portfolio would be an acceptable mechanism of providing this evidence.

The third drive for portfolio development is revalidation for doctors. There has been much speculation as to what form revalidation will take. The General Medical Council has now suggested that a portfolio could provide a framework for evidence to an external review process in support of revalidation.[3]

The Toolbox for Portfolio Development is a guide written for all members of the primary healthcare team (doctors, nurses, practice managers, receptionists and professions allied to medicine) who are willing and prepared to learn from their work. It addresses the needs of each individual as well as the PHCT as a whole.

The material and templates provided allow a process of self-discovery by increasing self-awareness, which should help you develop your potential. The resulting portfolio will not only provide you with a process of learning but also a record of your learning experiences. Through the process of reflection, you will be able to identify your strengths and weaknesses and address your learning needs accordingly.

Portfolios can be difficult to conceive. Many wonder what a portfolio should look like and want to know where to start. The toolbox aims to deal with these difficulties by creating a framework through which learning activity can be encouraged and recorded. It provides guidance and suggestions only and it is for each person to customise it for their own use. You may find some of the templates useful, or you may wish to develop your own. Some may be applicable to some PHCT members and not to others. The important point is that through regular reflection on your work, you will be developing your potential and attending to your professional development.

The Toolbox for Portfolio Development is divided into four parts. Part One addresses the theory behind portfolio learning and how the toolbox can work for you. Chapter 1 begins with an introduction to how we can learn 'on the job' and looks at the importance of reflection in learning and the processes involved. Chapter 2 explains how the portfolio, and in particular the toolbox, can contribute to personal and professional development. Chapter 3 explains the importance of identifying learning needs and describes the rationale behind personal education plans. Chapters 4 and 5 look at how support and help with learning can be provided in primary care. The processes of learning can be strengthened by the use of a 'helper'. The helper's role is to stand back and be objective, act like a mirror, and challenge any assumptions that you have made. The process of learning in primary healthcare cannot occur unless there is a culture of learning within the workplace and the organisation and this is explored in Chapter 5. Chapter 6 provides some tips on time management and on keeping a portfolio and the final chapter explores how learning and keeping a portfolio can contribute to clinical governance.

Part Two provides you with an opportunity to complete a personal and practice profile. The personal profile has also incorporated relevant sections for the revalidation of doctors.

Part Three (Sections A–D) provides you with a series of templates, which will guide you through the process of reflection. By completing these templates, you will not only have engaged in the process of learning but also have a product or record of your achievements. Sections A and B provide examples of templates of learning from your patients, from other professionals and from your personal life experiences. All are valid to your development as a health professional within primary care. Much of the material in these sections will contribute towards the development of clinical governance. Section D explains and provides help in demonstrating how the templates can contribute towards clinical governance.

Part Four contains appendices, which you may find useful. Appendix 1 is a suggested proforma for a teacher portfolio. Appendix 2 demonstrates how the toolbox can contribute to revalidation for doctors and Appendix 3 has useful names, addresses and websites.

The issues of health quality can only begin to be tackled when individual members of the primary healthcare team work and learn together. *The Toolbox for Portfolio Development* addresses not only the learning needs of individual members of PHCTs, but also those of the team as a collective unit. The process of each individual keeping a portfolio that addresses their own learning needs as well as those of the team will help to create a culture of learning. An environment in which learning (and particularly learning from experience) is valued and recognised should create a strong, committed team. As a consequence the PHCT can develop its potential and be able to address improvements in healthcare.

In a book promoting self-direction and autonomy in learning, it would appear contrary to these principles to create a framework that might seek to straitjacket learners through the use of templates covering a variety of learning activities. It is precisely because people do have difficulty in conceiving their portfolio and appear to want help in starting, that the templates have been created.

Some people may find it useful to work with the templates, whilst others will wish to design new ones or add their own. *The Toolbox for Portfolio Development* can offer flexibility because the suggested templates contained within the second part of the toolbox are meant only as a guide. It is designed to improve learning through a process of systematic recording of an individual's or group's experiences and reflections. It addresses the three important issues:

- continuing professional development
- revalidation
- clinical governance.

The resulting product should:

- provide a log of the learning and development
- demonstrate how an individual and a team have developed their potential

- provide a log of how clinical governance has been addressed.

Finally, *The Toolbox for Portfolio Development*, like any portfolio, is not a static document and should be in the process of development and change. It should be customised and each PHCT member may wish to modify and adapt the toolbox for his or her own use. Above all, it is important that the toolbox is 'owned' by each individual.

Part One

Portfolio-based learning in primary care

Chapter 1

How adults learn best: the importance of reflection

'Experience is not what happens to you . . . it is what you do with what happens to you.' Aldous Huxley

'Learning without thought is labour lost, thought without learning is perilous.' Confucius

---

Much of the work carried out on how adults learn suggests that it is important for them to take the initiative and to assume control of their education. Learning is best achieved when learners are able to choose what they learn and how they learn.[4] Evaluating what has been achieved and having an opportunity to apply the learning are also important. In other words, it is essential to be active in all stages of the learning process.

Time for reflection is considered an important part of any learning experience. If you are exposed to one new experience after another, without an opportunity for reflection, then any learning achieved is short-lived or lost. A period of thinking through or reflection is necessary to make sense of any experience and enables you to learn from the experience.[5] Making time available for reflection is an important precursor to learning. This process of learning has been called 'learning on action' or 'action learning'.[6] It is a continuous process based on the strong relationship between reflection and action, which leads to learning.

Learning on action or experience can be expressed in the form of a four-stage continuous cycle adapted from Kolb:[7]

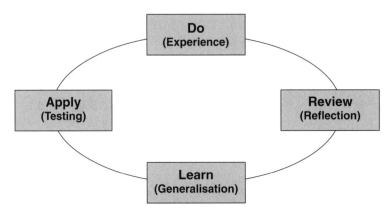

The learning process

The four-stage cycle needs to be completed for effective learning to take place. A balance needs to be achieved between doing and thinking or reflecting. It is not sufficient to just do or think. You need to do both and link the two together for learning to occur.[8] The rest of the cycle involves relating your new learning to what you already know and finally, applying this new knowledge to your work.

Reflection is crucial to the cycle. For example, it is not enough just to attend a lecture or a course; you need to provide time to think about what you have heard or experienced. If you do not go through this process of reflection, the essence of the lecture and any new learning or application to your work may be lost. You may remember some things immediately after a lecture, but unless you have an opportunity to reflect and think about what you have heard, your memory may be short-lived. To make the most of any experience, you will need to make time to think through the event and see if you can make some sense out of it. This discipline will lead to the retention of new knowledge or understanding, the development of a new skill or a change in behaviour.[5]

Creating time for reflection may involve making notes about the lecture or discussing it with a colleague. Alternatively, writing a short summary of the salient points may be useful. It helps to try to link what you already know about the subject to your new learning. You can then look at what you have learnt and examine how this might affect and influence the way you work.

Attending lectures is not the only way of learning. You can learn a great deal from your everyday work. Work should be and is a rich source of learning. You can learn either on your own, through reading, through formal or informal discussion with colleagues or through your work with patients. It is almost a cliché to say that you can learn most from your patients but this is very true. The potential for learning from everyday work experiences may not always be fully maximised. To make the most of these learning opportunities there is a need to acknowledge this potential for learning and to create time for reflection. This should ensure learning is effective and not short-lived.

If you have the misfortune to make a serious mistake in the course of your work, it will probably stay in your memory. If other people know of your mistake this may increase your embarrassment. Because of the seriousness of the mistake and the embarrassment it has caused, you may be forced into reflection. You might have to talk to other people at work about the mistake and confide and share your distress with people close to you. It may be difficult for you to avoid thinking about your error. Because you have been forced into reflecting and thinking through your experience, it is very unlikely that you will repeat the same mistake. If, however, the mistake is small and has little consequence, and does not become known to others, you may not be forced into a period of reflection. The mistake may indicate a lack of knowledge or skill and you may resolve to address this learning need or deficiency and have very good intentions of doing so. But other things occupy your mind and you may forget about your learning deficiency. Some time later, because you have not adequately reflected upon it or addressed your learning need, you may find that you repeat the same mistake.

Reflection is not just about thinking. It involves several different processes and sometimes the word 'critical' is added before 'reflection' to denote the importance of the processes. Critical reflection 'is concerned with developing the ability to assess both explicit and implicit claims, so as to determine what I ought to do, or which claim I ought to accept, on the basis of good reasons for that decision – rather than on the basis of force, chance or custom'.[9] It involves 'our recognising the assumptions underlying our beliefs and behaviours. It means we can give justifications for our ideas and actions. Most importantly, perhaps, it means we try to judge the rationality of these justifications'.[10]

Critical reflection has been described as a three-stage process:[5]

1 Remembering and recollecting the learning experience

The first stage involves revisiting the experience or event. Remembering the potential learning experience may be achieved by reading through any notes you made at the time or soon after. Relating it to someone else can also help you recollect the experience. This is an important process because sometimes, by verbalising and recounting what happened, details emerge or are remembered that might otherwise have been lost. Although at this stage the recollection is purely descriptive, it may prompt subconscious or poorly remembered events to be described, leading to the development of a different insight into the experience.

2 Thinking about how the experience made you feel

The experience or event may have resulted in positive or negative feelings. It is important to explore these feelings because unless they are addressed and acknowledged, useful learning is not achieved. This process involves:

- looking at the positive feelings (what aspects made you feel challenged, motivated, excited, stimulated, supported)
- looking at the negative feelings (what aspects made you feel uncomfortable, threatened, de-valued).

It is all too easy sometimes to focus on the negative feelings and this may only lead to de-motivation. It is important to start from a position of strengths and what you do or have done well. It is only then that you can begin to look at how you can do better.

3 Re-evaluating the experience

Having gone through the first two processes, you will now need to think about the value and potential application of your new learning. This involves:

- associating and integrating what you may have learnt with your previous knowledge and experience
- validating or checking out the newly gained knowledge or skill in your own mind to see whether it would work in practice
- translating it into a conclusion, a learning outcome or an action plan.

To be effective, this conscious process of critical reflection requires a structured approach. It often involves making notes, jotting down what you did or felt. How often does it happen that a learning need may be discovered during the course of a day and is not addressed and forgotten? You may find a gap in your knowledge during the course of your work and write down your learning need on a piece of paper with good intentions to address the problem later. But the piece of paper may be lost or, if looked at some time later, its relevance may be obscure. In order to learn from your everyday experiences, a system or a structure needs to be developed to ensure you do not lose the potential for learning.

To achieve effective learning in your work, two things need to be created: *time* and a process that brings about and strengthens reflection: a *portfolio*.

Time

Time is not easy to create. There are many tasks to complete during the course of each working day and often there is no time to address even these tasks, let alone additional ones. Because of the lack of time, there may be a tendency to respond to everyday events as they happen, often spontaneously and perhaps without too much thought. You may have to work extra hours or may take work home in order to keep abreast. Under these working conditions, reflection and analysis tend to be reserved only for a crisis or a significant event. How can time be found during the course of a day to reflect?

The answer lies with prioritising and according the time for reflection the importance it deserves. If you have many tasks to complete in the course of a day, you need to learn to plan how you can make the best use of your time. The secret to time management is planning, planning and planning! Try to create a regular or fixed time each week to plan and reflect. Learning and work should become interwoven, rather than separate experiences. Further tips on time management are provided in Chapter 6.

By recognising that a great deal of learning can occur within your own sphere of work, you may be able to save time by not travelling to other places for your learning. Allowing time for reflection and keeping a portfolio will address many varied needs and could actually save you a great deal of time. For example, a portfolio could not only provide evidence of your continuing professional development, but also address the issues of clinical governance and revalidation.

Portfolio

A portfolio is a record of your learning experiences which provides evidence of reflection and learning. A learning activity is not in itself evidence of learning. This is the error of the PGEA (for doctors) which rewards attendance at learning activities rather than the actual learning itself. Attending an educational event is not necessarily evidence of learning. Your mind may have been on other things and your attention span short. Alternatively, you may have acquired some new knowledge but did not put it into practice. Therefore whenever you engage in any learning activity, it is important that you provide yourself with an opportunity to reflect upon the educational experience. An attempt should be made to identify the learning outcome. For example, this might be a reinforcement of existing knowledge, new knowledge gained, a new skill acquired or a change in attitude. All learning activities and their outcomes should be recorded in your portfolio.

The portfolio also provides an opportunity for you to discover your learning needs. It allows you to plan how you might address these needs. It can be the focus to record the implementation of learning activities, their outcomes and applications and provide you with a record of your educational achievements.

This process of learning has been called portfolio-based learning.[11,12] Portfolio-based learning is both a process and a product. The process of keeping a portfolio (i.e. keeping records, making notes, and keeping a diary) engages you in reflection on the experience or learning activity. By keeping a portfolio, you will be providing yourself with a mechanism for reflecting and reinforcing learning. In addition, the portfolio will result in a product. By providing you with a log of your educational experiences, your learning and learning outcomes, it may, if desired, be submitted for accreditation or validation. It may also form part of an impressive curriculum vitae.

Portfolio-based learning enables you to focus on all your experiences. As you learn from your everyday experiences, you need to be able to recognise their learning potential. These may be related not only to your work but also to personal life experiences. There is an unnecessary artificial division between life and work experiences and learning. To a certain extent, attending courses or lectures may encourage this division and the misconception that learning is best achieved in educational institutions. Whilst attending educational events is a valuable way of learning and keeping up to date, it should not be the only way. In fact, many people experience problems in transferring learning gained from an educational event back into the work situation. So effective learning can occur not only in the workplace but also through personal life experiences.

Portfolio-based learning puts you in charge of your own education and enables you to tailor your learning programme to your needs and your own preferred learning style. Your continuing development need not therefore be from one type of educational activity. Contributions to your portfolio could be from a variety of activities that reflect your preferred method of learning. Examples of entries into your portfolio could include audits, lectures attended, notes, learning needs identified and addressed, patient satisfaction analysis, appraisals, personal education plans and so on.

Sharing the portfolio with a helper can significantly enhance the process of reflection. A helper (or mentor) could be anyone – a colleague or even the PHCT. A helper should be objective and may not only reinforce reflection but should help to ensure that the process is rigorous and well focused. For further details on the role of the helper see Chapter 4.

Chapter 2

What is *The Toolbox for Portfolio Development*?

'I have learnt throughout my life as a composer, chiefly through my mistakes and pursuits of false assumptions, not by my experience to founts of wisdom and knowledge.' Igor Stravinsky

'Experience is the name everyone gives to their mistakes.' Oscar Wilde

The Toolbox for Portfolio Development is an approach to learning that allows you to be in charge of your own education and professional development at a pace that suits you. It creates a framework through which all learning activity can be recorded. The resulting portfolio will provide a collection of all that you and/or your practice has done and experienced and the learning that has arisen from the activity.

Much of learning can be spontaneous and elusive. You may get a sudden insight into a problem, a flash of inspiration, an intuitive understanding. Unless this is captured, and recorded in the portfolio, it may be lost.[5] Therefore the portfolio may contain anything that can demonstrate the learning. The list is endless and you can enter anything you wish into your portfolio. It could include writing, photographs or videos. Most importantly the portfolio should contain your reflections. Some possible examples include:

- notes or handouts from meetings or courses attended
- articles or papers that have been read and your interpretations of them
- activities completed (e.g. audit, setting guidelines, designing protocols)
- consultation logs or videos and their analysis

- identification of learning needs
- projects
- case descriptions
- examples of learning with and from other health professionals
- workload logs
- patient satisfaction analysis
- examples of patient complaints and how they have been addressed.

One of the factors hindering the development of portfolios has been that, to many, portfolios are difficult to conceive. They appear nebulous and ethereal. Concerns are also expressed about how to begin developing a portfolio. Many have wondered what a portfolio should look like. The suggestion that a portfolio is whatever you wish to make it and that it can be designed and developed to suit your own needs has not proved helpful to most people.

The Toolbox for Portfolio Development aims to deal with these difficulties by creating a framework through which all learning activity can be recorded. The framework is provided by learning activity templates to help record learning. A template creates a structure by which you can record your activity and log the learning from the activity. It provides a mechanism for reflecting on the experience.

In primary care, learning from experience, through reflective practice, may be considered to arise from three sources. These are:

- what we learn from patients
- what we learn from other health professionals, either directly or indirectly
- what we learn from personal life experiences.

For each of these sources, examples of suggested learning activity templates are provided in Part Three. Because what we learn from these three sources contributes to our personal and professional development, this influences the quality of healthcare we provide. As clinical governance concerns the quality of healthcare, there is an inevitable overlap between education and development and clinical governance. A fourth section in Part Three addresses the issue of clinical governance.

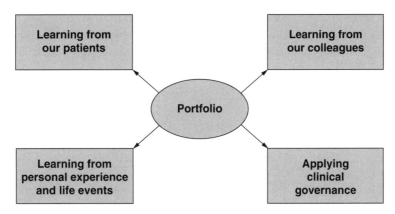

The toolbox for portfolio development

Learning from patients

Whether you are a doctor, nurse or receptionist, you have contact with patients. Patients, of course, tend to present to us during illness and we can and do learn a great deal from them. Although illnesses may be the same, people are not and how one person reacts to an illness may be quite different from how another person reacts. Therefore you can learn not only about the illness or disease but also about human development, human psychology and the human condition. People need healthcare at different stages of their lives and at different stages of their human development. They may present when they are happy or sad, they may be in good health or they may be ill. You cannot fail to learn something of human development and of human suffering through the interaction with patients. Through your experiences and how you react to and interpret them, you may develop an understanding and an insight. This can only help your professional development.

Learning from colleagues

You also learn from your colleagues with whom you work, those within your own profession and in allied professions. You can learn from your colleagues through direct contact with them either in formal or informal meetings or exchanges. You also have indirect contact with your colleagues either through correspondence or reading books, articles or papers. By sharing your experiences with your colleagues and by listening to and observing colleagues with different experiences, you can gain valuable learning.

Learning from personal life experiences

You may also learn from your own personal life experiences and this is no less valid. You experience similar life events to those your patients experience, such as bereavement, loss, having a family, bringing up children, looking after aged parents. All of these may contribute to how you react and relate to patients who have similar experiences. Of course you should not judge patients by the way you would respond in similar circumstances. But if you share similar life experiences, this will help you help your patients. You don't have to experience a bereavement to be able to support a patient with a similar experience, but if you have been through a bereavement, this may provide you with greater insight and understanding of your patient's difficulties and will help you empathise with them.

Anything that demonstrates learning from these significant life events may contribute to the portfolio. Evidence may be written or visual (photographs, videos). They may be other areas within this section that may also include learning from culture. For example, art, reading, the media, film, theatre, radio or television can provide us with an insight into human psychology and the human condition. This inevitably will influence and impinge on your work.

Applying clinical governance

Clinical governance is about health professionals being accountable for setting, maintaining and monitoring performance standards. It is inclusive, involving all healthcare staff (practice managers, receptionists, PAMs as well as nurses and doctors). Although clinical governance concerns accountability, if this alone is allowed to drive its implementation, it will be perceived as a threat. But if clinical governance is viewed as part of a programme of education, training and continuing development, it is more likely to lead to the stated goal of improving quality. There is much overlap between learning from experience and maintaining standards. Many of the templates provided within the toolbox can contribute to clinical governance.

Examples of the learning activity templates provided cover all four areas. By completing many of them, you will be addressing these areas that are pertinent to your learning from your work.

The learning activity templates are for guidance only. You do not need to follow or complete them slavishly. It is important to stress that the templates aim to be flexible and not prescriptive. For those who experience difficulty in starting their portfolio, the toolbox provides examples of things that could be included in your portfolio. You may find it useful to work with the templates, or you may not wish to be compartmentalised and would prefer to design your own learning templates. The toolbox is principally concerned with providing a framework through which you can demonstrate your learning and your continuing professional development.

A quality health service is dependent on efficient and effective teamwork. Administrative staff should not only be involved in organisational and practice management issues but they also have a crucial and important role in the delivery of all aspects of healthcare, be it acute or chronic. Their experience and observations may be quite different to clinical staff and they are able to make valuable contributions to the improvement of clinical care. A PHCT can gain a great deal from sharing their experiences and learning from and with each other. The principles of learning apply to everybody and the toolbox is applicable to all members of the PHCT. Most of the templates will certainly be applicable to clinical staff (doctors, nurses, health visitors, PAMs) and many will also be applicable to administrative staff (receptionists, practice managers).

Many of the exercises may be carried out alone. Assessing yourself means holding up a mirror so that you can stand back and observe how you interact with people and your work. If you are able to share your thoughts with another colleague or colleagues, the exercises may become more useful. Another colleague or helper can stand back and be objective and challenge you regarding any assumptions that you have.

First and foremost the toolbox is a learning tool. The process of working through, reflecting and keeping a record of your experiences will improve your learning. As mentioned in Chapter 1, the portfolio not only provides you with a process of learning but also with a product. The recording of your experiences will demonstrate how your learning has been achieved and how you have developed your potential as a professional person. A portfolio will therefore provide you with a log of all your development. But there are many other uses; for example it:

- may help discover your further learning needs. It can identify any gaps in your knowledge or skills
- can contribute to the way you and your practice deal with clinical governance issues from audit to clinical risk management to healthcare provision and so on
- can provide an important record of in-house training and multi-professional learning
- can provide satisfactory evidence of continuing professional development
- might contribute to the process of revalidation (for nurses, it will for example be acceptable to the UKCC)
- can be used as a record of work experience and therefore contribute to further professional aspirations
- will recognise your achievements and your successes
- will identify your further development through the setting of action plans
- will encourage lifelong learning.

Chapter 3

Identifying learning needs and personal education plans

'Learners need to . . . write off their mistakes as experience . . . We change by exploration not by tracing well known paths . . . We start our learning with uncertainties and doubts, with questions to be resolved. We grow older wondering who we will be and what we will do . . . If we cannot live with these uncertainties we will not learn and change will always be an unpleasant surprise.' C Handy

Keeping a portfolio will help you to identify your learning needs. These are gaps in your knowledge, skills and attitudes that need addressing in order to perform your work efficiently. They are the gaps between your current and desired proficiencies. To determine your learning needs, you can try and identify your own or others can identify them with you.

Identifying your own needs is subjective and can be difficult. Because of this your assessment may not be truly accurate. Self-assessment of learning needs makes certain assumptions. It assumes that you are able to:

- expose the learning need during the course of your work
- recognise it as a gap in your proficiency

and finally

- that you are able to be honest enough with yourself to admit it.

Assessing your own learning needs can be a powerful and important tool in your continuing development. As long as you can remain aware of the above assumptions and keep them in your mind, you will find it a useful technique. Many of the learning activity templates should help you to identify your own learning needs. An objective and perhaps more accurate method of identifying your learning needs would be to enlist the help of another person or persons. Ideally, you should begin by trying to identify your own needs first and then you could check out your assumptions with your colleagues or your mentor. This could help confirm or validate your own assessment.

The Johari window was described by Joseph Luft and Harry Ingram in 1955.[13] It can graphically illustrate the difference between assessing yourself and obtaining other peoples' viewpoints. The window can be seen as representing you and what you know and don't know about yourself, what other people know and don't know about you. The window is divided into four panes of glass.

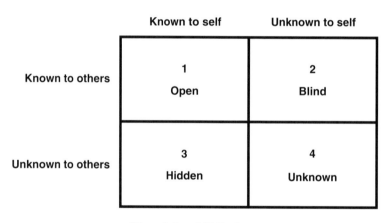

The Johari Window

The first pane represents what you know about yourself and what other people know about you. It may relate to facts, behaviour or feelings about you. It is public knowledge and known to all. It represents the open part of your character.

The second pane represents what you do not know about yourself but what other people know about you. It may, for example, relate to your behaviour or the way you respond in certain situations that you may be unaware of. It represents the blind part of your character.

The third pane represents what you know about yourself but do not wish to share with other people. Other people have no knowledge of these secrets. They may be secrets about your behaviour or feelings that you do not wish to disclose or become known. It represents the hidden part of your character.

The fourth pane represents what you do not know about yourself and what others do not know either. This unknown part of you may influence the way you behave or think but you are unaware of this. It represents the unknown part of your character.

In terms of your learning needs, the first pane represents what you are prepared to admit you know and don't know. Other people would agree with your assessment. So this pane represents your proficiencies from your perspective and those of others. The third pane represents what you know you don't know, i.e. the gaps in your proficiency which you are unwilling to share with other people. This might be because you are embarrassed about the gaps in your knowledge and you wish to hide them. Nevertheless you are aware of them. They represent what you consider you know or what you know you don't know. So this pane represents your proficiencies from your own perspective only and is not known to others.

The second and fourth panes represent your learning needs of which you are unaware. You may not know that you are performing badly on one aspect of your job, because you lack the knowledge or skill that you require to perform that aspect of your job well. To other people, your ignorance or your substandard performance may be apparent (second pane). Alternatively, even other people may not be aware that you are performing badly. They, like you, may be unaware of your learning needs (fourth pane).

Learning needs can be considered to be of two main types: perceived and true. The panes 1 and 3 in the Johari window represent your learning needs from your perspective. They are your perceived learning needs of which you are aware that may become true learning needs through an objective independent assessment. So panes 2 and 4 are not your perceived needs but may well be your true needs.

The Johari window panes are not static and knowledge and information about you can move from one pane to another. You can gain insight into your learning needs not only by becoming more open and honest with other people but also through the way you receive feedback about yourself. For example, if you share your perceived needs with others through disclosure, you will obtain a more objective insight into your true needs. By revealing that part of your hidden area (pane 3) you are becoming more open. By sharing your hidden area with others and being open to feedback, you will also be reducing your blind area (pane 2).

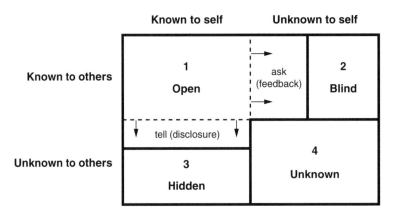

The Johari Window

Finally by being more open and sharing with others you may begin to get new insight into yourself and thereby discover new learning needs that were previously in your unknown area (pane 4).

Personal education (development or action) plan

Once a need is identified it is useful and important to say how you intend to tackle this learning need. By doing this, you are not only putting yourself in charge of your own learning but you are also making a commitment or a 'contract' with yourself to address the learning need. A personal education (development or action) plan or learning contract is a structured approach that is a valuable way of formalising your intended programme of learning and also helps to maximise your learning. It is an agreement to undertake a learning exercise and has a number of stages[4]

What do you need to learn?

This is the first stage and involves finding out your learning need. This represents the gap between where you are now and where you would like to be. It may represent a gap in your knowledge or skills that you need to rectify in order for you to perform your job more effectively.

What do you hope to achieve?

Having identified your learning need you should state clearly what you hope to achieve (your objectives) and what you would like your learning outcome to be.

How will you do it? What resources will you need?

This involves you identifying what help you will need to achieve your learning and the form the learning will take. For example, will you attend a lecture or a course or will you learn through doing? Will you need the help of a person or a group?

How will you be able to show what you have learnt or accomplished?

This stage involves you identifying how you intend to show evidence of your learning achievement. What will this evidence look like? It could, for example, be an achievement of your objectives. In addition, you will also need to provide evidence of how you plan to put your new learning into practice. How will the success be judged (what are the criteria?) and by whom (how will it be validated?)?

Review your plan

Ideally you should share your plan with someone else with a more objective assessment (a friend, a colleague or colleagues) allowing you to make any changes after discussion. This could be formal or informal but is useful because of the insights obtained with an objective overview of the plan. It will, for example, clarify whether it is realistic and achievable.

Carry out your plan

Now you embark on your learning exercise. Your plan should be flexible to allow you to make changes in the light of your progress.

Evaluate what you have learnt

Having completed your learning exercise, you will need to evaluate what you have been able to achieve against your objectives and the criteria you set yourself at the start.

The whole process of writing out an education plan might seem unnecessary and tedious but the actual involvement in the process helps to put you in control of your own learning. This control means that you are more likely to enjoy it and to make a success of your own learning. It offers another opportunity for reflection that helps to reinforce learning.

Determining learning needs and devising personal education plans can be carried out either by an individual or a group. A PHCT could determine their learning needs as a group of people working together. They could then go on to formulate a practice education (or development) plan. For example, a PHCT could meet and decide how they as a group could improve on the healthcare of a specific problem (e.g. people with diabetes). Alternatively, they could begin to address standards (e.g. those set by NSFs).

Through discussion a learning need for the practice and its PHCT as a whole may be identified. The PHCT could then go on to devise the practice education plan. A structure to help the group identify learning needs might be a SWOT exercise. SWOT is an acronym for:

Strengths – what are you doing well, what are you proud of, and what have you been able to achieve?

Weaknesses – what aren't you so good at, what could you do better?

Opportunities – what opportunities are available to help you develop and improve?

Threats – what is preventing you from achieving your goal(s)?

The SWOT analysis can be used as a framework for beginning to examine improvements within the practice with the purpose of introducing change which will hopefully lead to improvement in quality of care. The exercise can be carried out by an individual or a group, each area being tackled in turn.

The process is normally carried out through a brainstorming exercise. A flip chart presenting the areas in four boxes allows the group to see at a glance the suggestions as they are volunteered.

Strengths	Weaknesses
Opportunities	Threats

SWOT analysis

By working through an exercise such as the SWOT analysis, a practice can identify their learning needs and the factors that would help or prevent them from addressing these needs. Of equal importance is that the team will have also been able to identify what they do well. Starting from strengths and acknowledging and celebrating them will not only enable the team to tackle the areas that need developing, but it will also help to cement team bonding. At the end of the exercise, it is possible to draw upon a list of issues that need to be addressed.

Chapter 4

What is the role of a 'helper' in keeping a portfolio?

'Everyone who makes it has a mentor.' *Harvard Business Review*

Keeping a portfolio will help reflection and strengthen learning. Sometimes it is necessary to stand back from the work you do and obtain a more objective view. This is difficult to do alone and it may be necessary to seek the help of a colleague or a group. Another person can act as a mirror and see things in a different way. By challenging your assumptions and conclusions, reflections and interpretations, this 'helper' can provide you with a different perspective. Their view of your experience may be valuable. Alternatively, he or she may help to confirm your original conclusion, which is equally valid and important.

A helper's role can be:

- to help with any difficulties
- to be supportive and encouraging
- to help identify resources
- to be challenging
- to praise
- to remind the learner of their strengths and weaknesses.

Helpers have been called mentors and their role in the personal and professional development of adults has increased in significance in recent years. The original

Mentor in Greek mythology was a wise counsellor, father figure and role model to Telemachus, whose father, Odysseus, was busy with the Trojan wars. The concept of a mentor was resurrected in the 1980s, when it found a place in business, and subsequently mentors were used in the continuing education of a variety of professions.[14]

It is not difficult to see why the concept of mentoring has become popular. The major influence has been the development of the current theories and principles of effective learning. Learning is best achieved if learners are allowed to take control of their own learning and are active in the process of learning (learner-centred education). In addition, there has been a shift towards learning within the workplace and the recognition of the need to encourage reflection in action. This move towards learner-centred education has led to the learner becoming more self-directed. Being in charge of your own learning will inevitably increase demands, necessitating the need for some sort of support. Support would seek to avoid the learner being isolated and provide help, advice and challenge. This would promote self-confidence, self-esteem and self-awareness. One mechanism for learning support can be provided through a mentor.

The mentor is a facilitator, encouraging learners to set their own strategies for learning. He or she will help the learner to identify resources for their learning, to help with any difficulties that arise and to help them discover and challenge their own solutions. The mentor has a key role in helping the learner reflect critically on their experience and explore different perspectives. Above all the mentor needs to be able to offer pastoral care. This involves providing help and support, and encouragement.

Who can act as a helper or mentor? The answer is anybody with the necessary qualities and skills. They need to be able to be genuine and honest which means they are true to themselves and to others. They should not hide or be defensive. They also need to respect the person they are helping. Respect means being able to value and accept the individual as a human being. Rogers called this 'unconditional positive regard'.[15] Showing respect and being genuine are seen as the core values in a mentoring relationship, but there are other important skills that are related to good communication.

Listening is one of the most important skills. It is an active process which is not only about hearing what the other person is saying. It involves a physical and a psychological presence where the listener gives their undivided attention. Having an awareness of the verbal and the non-verbal message and any inconsistencies in what is being said is important. Empathic listening and reflection of feeling can be powerful. It involves the listener rejecting any prejudices they might have, and putting themselves in the learner's position, providing an understanding from their perspective. Acceptance of statements at face value will lead to a collusive relationship. Understanding can be improved through probe and challenge and this should not compromise the need for the mentor to show respect.

Whilst being mentored, you must in turn respect your mentor, who may be a colleague from work or unrelated to work, and have trust regarding issues such as confidentiality. You may have reservations regarding sharing your experiences with a colleague or a group that you work with every day, or concerns regarding confidentiality, or doubt whether they can be truly honest and avoid colluding with you. These issues need to be addressed and explored with your mentor. If you are still concerned about these issues then a mentor from outside your workplace may be the answer.

There are various models of mentoring. Reviewing the literature, Maynard and Furlong described three distinct historical models.[16] The **apprenticeship model** dates back to Aristotle. Here learning is best achieved through supervised practice and through the observation of an experienced practitioner. It is also known as the 'sitting with Nellie' approach. The learner learns through role modelling, and the mentor provides interpretation and solutions to problems that work in practice. The **competency model** is similar to that of a coach or trainer. The mentor may have a list of predetermined competencies and through a systematic process of observation and feedback, the learner develops their potential. The third model is the **reflective practitioner model**. This involves a significant shift away from the two above. It involves the mentor moving from role model, coach or trainer to co-enquirer. The relationship is less hierarchical and the intention is to promote critical reflection.

There are other different models of mentoring.[17] There is no reason why two people may not mentor each other. Again the issue of possible collusion will need to be addressed and recognised. A mentor may also provide support for a group of people, for example the practice team, or alternatively a group (the practice team) may mentor an individual. The model you choose will depend on your preferences and the availability of a suitable mentor or mentors.

Chapter 5

The primary healthcare team as a learning organisation

'We learn best from experience but we never directly experience the consequences of many of our important decisions.' P Senge

'We learn through experience and experiencing and no one teaches anyone. This is as true for the infant moving from kicking to crawling to walking as it is for the scientist with his equations. If the environment permits it, anyone can learn; and if the individual permits it, the environment will teach him everything it has to teach.' Viola Spolin

In the last few years, there have been increasing demands for providers of healthcare to be more accountable, and to ensure that all patients receive high quality care. The concept of clinical governance has emerged to respond to this need. Clinical governance (*see* Chapter 7) involves being accountable for setting, maintaining and monitoring performance standards in order to deliver high quality healthcare. It involves every member of the PHCT and each has an important and vital role to play within the team.

The ability of the PHCT to deliver high quality healthcare is dependent on the development of a culture that will support this. This is recognised in numerous government documents, where one keyword that is continually repeated is this notion of culture. *A First Class Service: quality in the new NHS* states that the key to improvement in quality of healthcare will involve *'creating a culture'* or supporting *'a change in culture'*.[2] It goes on to state that primary care will need to be '*underpinned by a culture that values lifelong learning*' and that this involves a '*major cultural change for everyone*'. Culture must be considered to be important but what is the meaning of culture as applied to a practice team? How can a culture begin to value lifelong learning?

The culture of an organisation is not easy to define and the implication from the above is that it is something that can be produced, developed and modified. Culture can be seen as an environment, which is '*shared between colleagues in an organisation, including shared beliefs, attitudes, values and norms of behaviour. Thus, organisational culture is reflected by a common sense of the organisation that allows people to see situations and events in similar and distinctive ways. It is "the way things are done around here", as well as the way things are understood, judged and valued*'.[18]

A PHCT can be considered to be a NHS organisation with its own culture. It represents a group of healthcare colleagues working together, engaged in the process of delivering healthcare to its local population and community. It should be seen to be more than a collection of individuals working with a similar purpose. The individuals should be working together as a unit and as a team, valuing each other's contribution. Each individual member of the team has a different background, role and expertise. Instead of trying to search for similarities between individuals, the challenge is to examine the differences. The recognition and acknowledgement of these differences leads to valuing the individual within the team, which strengthens the team and its purpose.[19]

It has been accepted for many years that the delivery of good quality healthcare is best achieved through effective collaborative working between different disciplines and professions.[20] Through teamwork, the whole (the PHCT) becomes greater than the sum of the parts (the individual members). This is known as positive synergy.[18] The direct contrast to this results in negative synergy, where an organisation is hierarchical and fragmented. In order to achieve this positive synergy, the concept or the culture of a learning organisation needs to be established.

A learning organisation is one: '*that facilitates learning of all its members and continually transforms itself*'.[21] It is an organisation where its members '*continually expand their capacity to create the results they truly desire, where new expansive patterns of thinking are nurtured, where collective aspiration is set free, and where people are continually learning to learn together*'.[22]

To develop a learning organisation, a number of values, beliefs and attitudes should be fostered. An individual member's contribution is valued and their need to learn and develop recognised. It is accepted that learning occurs independently and collectively within the workplace. Investment in learning is a high priority for a learning organisation. It encourages learning from mistakes and learning from successes. To become a learning organisation, an environment of trust and openness needs to be developed and encouraged, an environment that is free of blame or shame.

The difference between the factors that promote and inhibit a learning organisation can be summarised in the table below:

Factors facilitating the development of a learning organisation	Factors inhibiting the development of a learning organisation
Reflective – thinking and planning recognised as important	Bureaucratic – too focused on processes and service delivery
Active encouragement of further learning	Reluctance to provide time for or invest in training
Embraces change and risk-taking	Reluctance to institute change – maintains traditional approaches
Recognises value of workplace and action learning, providing time	Work is for work and time is money
Open democratic culture – empowerment of members	Closed hierarchical culture – members toe the line; hidden personal agendas
Learning from experience recognised – successes celebrated and lessons learnt from mistakes	Learning from experience not recognised – successes ignored; mistakes not tolerated and not seen as useful for learning
Fosters individual and collective team learning	Learning in isolation
Service provision responsive to patients and their needs	Service provision not driven by patients' needs
Strong supportive team	Team fragmented

Once a PHCT becomes a learning organisation, it can begin to address the issues of improvement in the quality of healthcare. By being a learning organisation, a climate is created that nurtures learning. As a consequence the team as a whole learns and develops. This 'cultural transformation' is a crucial outcome of a successful learning organisation.[23]

Creating and developing such a culture takes time. It requires considerable effort and commitment of all the individuals in a practice team. A leader or leaders may emerge to help drive the concept forward, and any hierarchical structures may need to be redefined. Open discussions with all members of the team are encouraged and ground rules negotiated and set. The result should be a more equal and democratic organisation, the features of which are:

- the establishment of good communication channels
- recognition of the value of teamwork and that the sum of the whole is greater than the sum of the parts
- acknowledgement of the value not only of working together but also of learning together
- promotion and encouragement of openness, trust and honesty
- fostering a 'no blame or shame' environment
- the recognition and addressing of tension between working and learning from work, by providing protected time for the latter.

The creation of such a culture requires resources and support. For many, the changes required are significant, involving not only changes to existing structures and processes but also shifts in attitudes. The whole process of change cannot happen overnight and will take time. Support may come from PCGs, PCTs, academic units or Royal Colleges. An external resource or facilitator may be helpful. Establishing such a culture is a necessary and vital precursor to improving the quality of care and addressing the issues of clinical governance and the NSFs. Whilst the efforts required are considerable, the benefits to the team and the patients will be worth the challenge.

Chapter 6

Tips on time management and on keeping a portfolio

'Well that's passed the time.'
'It would have passed in any case.'
'Yes, but not so rapidly.' Samuel Beckett

One of the difficulties often expressed by people who wish to keep a portfolio is that they do not have the time to spend reflecting and recording their experiences. For most, devoting time to this activity would seem to be an impossibility during a working day which is busy and occupied with regular tasks.

Working in the health service, you not only have responsibilities for your work but equally you are also accountable for the quality of service you provide. This means that you must undertake and demonstrate your own continuing education and professional development. This is your individual responsibility and that of your practice. Decisions regarding the importance that is attached to continuing education and development need to be made by both parties. If it is recognised as a priority, then it will be necessary to ensure that time is set aside during the course of a working week. Finding this time needs commitment and organisation.

Time is structured, unified and fixed. There are a fixed number of seconds in a minute, minutes in an hour, hours in a day. We all have the same amount of time but our perception of time is different, relative and individual. It can vary with our mood, our activity and with our enjoyment of the activity. So time can 'fly' when we are enjoying ourselves or 'drag' when we are bored. Time is a concept we value and, like money, can be lost, wasted or even created. We appreciate its value because we recognise that time can be 'wasted' or 'killed' in worthless activities. We also talk about 'creating' time. How can we 'create' time when it is a fixed unit? The answer lies in effective time management.

By acknowledging the concept of time management, we are accepting that time can be manipulated and controlled to our advantage. We can do this through planning how time will be used and by avoiding time-wasting activities. Whether we are employed or self-employed determines the extent to which we can control time. An employee will have a fixed schedule of activities but, even within this framework, it may be possible to have some degree of control. Protected time for continuing development may need to be negotiated. Time management, like learning, is personal and needs to be adjusted to the individual's own preferred style.

Some tips on time management are given opposite.

Having addressed time, another important issue that needs consideration is confidentiality. Ideally a portfolio should be a personal document. There is no right way of keeping a portfolio.[5] You should be able to insert things in your portfolio that you consider important and relevant to you and your development. But if the portfolio is for revalidation or clinical governance, then a tension may develop between the things that you wish to include in the portfolio and the things that the external revalidation body may wish to be included. You may have entered things in your portfolio that you feel are for your eyes only. Do not let this stop you from making entries. If there are items that are personal and confidential, you should be able to remove these if you need to show your portfolio to someone else. There is no reason why you cannot have more than one portfolio, each serving different purposes.

Your portfolio is not a static document – like you it changes and develops as you progress. Entries you make need to be dated. This will allow you to revisit them at a later date and make any additions as a result of developments or further reflections.

You are almost ready to start! First you need to decide how you will collect and store information for your portfolio. A system that allows you to add or remove documents easily such as a box file or a loose-leaf folder is ideal. It may be useful to have a mechanism for arranging the contents into sections – perhaps a set of dividers – so items can be easily retrieved. You may decide to keep your portfolio away from your workplace. If you do, you will need to think about how to record any learning needs or experiences as they happen. Keeping a small notebook

Tips on time management

(Adapted from Hayes[24])

- **Plan:** Plan your activities for the day/week. Make lists. Write out an action sheet – what has to be done and by when. Constantly review the sheet and tick off the items which have been addressed. If you have a large task to complete, divide it up into manageable sections, that way it will not seem insurmountable.

- **Prioritise:** Review your activities that you have planned and now prioritise them into:
  A = 'must do' (high priority)
  B = 'should do' (medium priority)
  C = 'nice to do' (low priority).
  You need to focus mainly on your 'A's. Set yourself a deadline in which to complete the tasks. Build in rewards and treat yourself if you like – they can be fun!

- **Deal with time wasters:** Avoid addressing a task more than once. Try and finish the task in hand (or if it's complex, break it up into different parts). If it's important, do it and complete it. If it's not an important task, why are you doing it? Make sure you handle each piece of paper once only – don't continually revisit it because you did not deal with it properly the first time, i.e. don't put things off. Avoid taking things on and overstretching yourself – give yourself permission to say 'no'. Rationalise the use of the telephone – it can cause a great deal of interruption and be a significant time waster.

- **Be tidy:** File things away and properly so that they can be easily retrieved and you do not waste time looking for them. Try and keep your desk clear.

- **Delegate:** Learn to delegate. Do not waste your time on tasks that others might be able to do equally well. You will need to delegate well and appropriately. Let go but make a distinction between delegating and abdicating – how much control will you need to retain?

handy for this purpose may help. It doesn't matter what system you use, it is more important that you find a system that works for you.

Some tips on keeping a portfolio follow.

Tips on keeping a portfolio

(Adapted from Boud, Keogh and Walker[5])

- Be frank and honest in your entries. 'Write it as it is, not as you would like it to be, nor as you think it should be.' Be open and sincere in what you record.

- Be positive and aggressive in approaching the portfolio. Do not dally round working out how you are going to do it; get down and do something. Let it flow, uncensored, and in whatever order it comes. It is very useful simply to write, and then reflect on what has been written. How often you make a portfolio entry is up to you, but try to write something in it at least weekly. It can be useful to set aside a fixed time every day to look at your portfolio.

- The portfolio is meant to be a workbook. Entries are to be worked through a number of times, and important aspects of them highlighted. Therefore, use underlining, circling, different coloured inks, and anything else that will draw out significant things.

- Be spontaneous, use your own words, and put your own name on things. Say what you feel and, if that makes you feel guilty, record that and work with it further. Do not be concerned about how you write. Do not look for style or literary eloquence, or worry that your writing does not seem to be great stuff.

- Take up issues that surface when you are working with the portfolio. Do not let other things take your attention. Focus on the important things, and do not waste time on trivialities.

- You should feel free to express yourself in whatever form you wish. Use diagrams, pictures, art, poems or whatever.

- Make regular times to write in the portfolio and a fixed time each week to reflect back on it. To use it to its fullest advantage, it is important to read over it frequently. It is not just writing in it that is important, but the continuing reflection on what has been written. One of the great enemies of the portfolio is procrastination.

- Record the experiences as soon as possible after they happen, and as fully as possible, when they are most fresh in your mind. You can refine your thoughts at a later date.

- You will need to develop a good filing system to ensure that you address the relevant areas in your portfolio. If you do not do this you could waste valuable time looking for documents.

Chapter 7

Addressing clinical governance

'We cannot change the human condition, but we can change the conditions under which humans work.' J Reason

The concept of clinical governance is defined as: 'a framework through which NHS organisations are accountable for continuously improving the quality of their services, safeguarding high standards by creating an environment in which excellence in clinical care will flourish'.[2]

The NHS is a public service and, like any other, it has to be accountable for the quality of its product – in this case, healthcare delivery. It needs to ensure that all patients receive high quality care. Clinical governance involves:

- every member of the primary healthcare team (practice managers, PAMs, receptionists, as well as nurses and doctors)
- providing high quality healthcare – this means setting standards of care and ensuring that they are delivered
- maintaining and monitoring the delivery of the standards of care
- improving on the quality of care
- accountability – not only doing the above but demonstrating that these issues of healthcare quality are being addressed.

For many in primary healthcare, these areas are, to a large extent, being continually addressed and clinical governance should build on existing activity. However, the implementation of clinical governance in primary care also demands a clear demonstration of it being addressed. A portfolio providing evidence of clinical governance could fulfil this need.

Although clinical governance concerns accountability, and is obligatory, it need not be seen as a threat or a chore. It should be viewed as part of a programme of continuing education, training and development. If approached in this manner, it is more likely to lead to the stated goal of improving quality. There is a large potential for overlap between clinical governance, revalidation and continuing education. To provide three packages of evidence demonstrating these concepts would be time-consuming and tedious. A single model might suffice and a portfolio should be able to do this.

In order to deliver the concept of clinical governance, the government has developed a number of structures. These have been represented by the diagram below:[2]

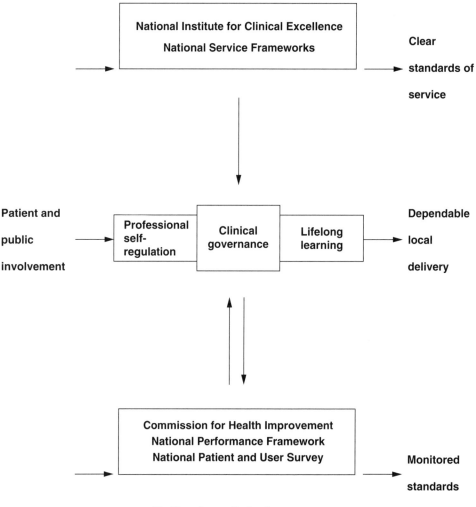

Delivering clinical governance

The *National Institute for Clinical Excellence (NICE)* was created in 1999 to:

- appraise the clinical evidence on existing treatments and new technologies
- develop and disseminate guidelines for all healthcare staff and patients
- provide support through the development of a range of audit methodologies and information on good practice.

NICE covers England and Wales only. Scotland is covered by the Scottish Health Technologies Assessment Centre (SHTAC).

The *National Service Frameworks (NSFs)* will:

- set national standards and define service models for a specific service or care group
- put in place programmes to support implementation
- establish performance measures against which progress within an agreed timescale will be measured.

The *Commission for Health Improvement (CHI)* will provide dissemination of clinical governance principles and independently scrutinise and monitor its implementation. It will also provide help and support where problems exist locally.

Not only will these bodies need to develop good communication channels between themselves but they will also require good communication and networking at:

- local level (NHS Trusts, health authorities, PCGs, PCTs and patient representative groups)
- regional level (regional offices)
- national level (Department of Health, Royal Colleges, academic units and other national representative groups).

Clinical governance covers a wide range of activities but the common denominator is high quality healthcare that is dependent on a number of factors. Many authors have referred to these factors as 'pillars' or the building blocks of clinical governance. These are:

- quality assurance, i.e. how good is the care provided?

- clinical audit i.e. how the care is monitored and analysed
- clinical effectiveness i.e. how efficient is the care provided?
- clinical risk management i.e. how safe is the care provided?
- staff and organisational development i.e. what is the quality and training of the staff and the organisation that provide that care?

Quality assurance

Quality assurance means a planned process in which healthcare is compared to predetermined standards, with the guarantee that changes will be implemented. These changes will be shown to have led to the desired improvements. Quality assurance encompasses various elements:

- it is a planned process, i.e. there is usually a programme rather than a 'one-off' exercise
- it compares performance against predetermined standards, i.e. how you perform against how you should perform (standards)
- it requires action (improvements) to be undertaken in the light of the comparison
- it requires a monitoring of the changes to ensure they have been implemented.

A standard is a measurable component of healthcare indicating an intended level of performance. The standards that you measure your performance against may be internally or externally based.

Internally-based standards

For example, these may be standards that you or your practice (the PHCT) decides. A variety of resources (articles, books, colleagues, experts, patients) can be used to help reach a clear definition of the standards.

Externally-based standards

These may be at a local level (determined by the HA or PCG), at a regional level (NHS Executive regional offices) or a national level (by NICE or NSFs). Local- and regional-based standards are to a large extent also guided by national standards. One example is the health improvement programme (HImP). This is a three-year plan determined locally, which aims to support the government's health programme. It is based on national guidelines but takes into account the local population and its needs. National guidance on standards of healthcare may come from NICE or NSFs as well as from academic units or Royal Colleges.

Examples of quality assurance are the national programmes for breast screening, cervical screening and immunisation.

Clinical audit

Audit can be seen as part of a programme of quality assurance and has become an acceptable part of general practice. If the quality of care provided is to improve, then it has to be the subject of continual audit.

Audit concerns the systematic process of critically analysing the quality of healthcare through measurement and evaluation. Its objective is to improve the quality of care provided through the introduction of change and monitoring the effects of this change. Certain key steps characterise the process and a successful audit is one that addresses all the steps. These will involve:

- defining of standards, or targets for good practice
- systematic gathering of the data concerning performance
- comparison of the results against the standards set
- identifying gaps in the performance
- identifying the action necessary to improve performance
- monitoring the effects of change in the service and repeating the audit.

Completing the audit cycle must include the last step, which is often neglected. Unless you go through the process of repeating the audit, i.e. collecting the data for a second time, you cannot be sure that audit has produced any change.

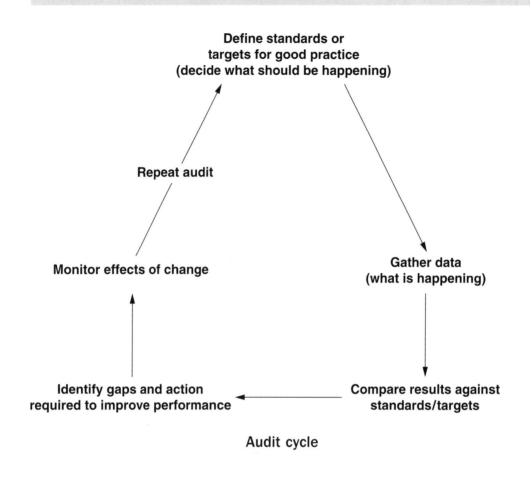

Audit cycle

Clinical effectiveness

It goes without saying that if clinical governance involves 'excellence in clinical care', then healthcare must not only be of high quality, it must be effective and efficient. Is the healthcare any good and is it cost-effective? This is clinical effectiveness.

A number of factors need to be considered if any organisation is to tackle the issue of clinical effectiveness. In order to produce effective and efficient healthcare, access to good quality data and results of research is needed. There needs to be an infrastructure of information technology that supports primary care and allows access, interpretation and dissemination of evidence-based medicine.

In recent years a number of useful resources have been set up. These are available in a variety of formats from documents from national institutions (e.g. NICE, NSF, NPCRDC) to journals or computer programs (e.g. *Bandolier, Effectiveness Matters,* Cochrane Library) to internet sites (CHAIN, CEBM, CGRDU). Resources need to be supported by opportunities for easy access within the working environment. Staff should be made aware of the resources available and how to access them.

Being aware of and accessing evidence-based material is only part of the equation to produce effective healthcare. There is also the need to create and facilitate a process of translating the evidence into practice.

Clinical risk management

Clinical risk management is about reducing or eliminating the potential for harm to patients and staff in healthcare organisations. The process requires an acknowledgement that errors can occur and are to a certain extent inevitable. Recognition of this may seem obvious but is necessary as a starting point. Humans are fallible and errors will always occur even in the most organised practice but through a systematic approach of review, reflection and action planning, errors can be minimised or avoided.

To embrace the concept of clinical risk management successfully, a practice should have established a climate of trust and openness and one that will avoid blame or shame (*see* Chapter 5). From this standpoint it can progress to capitalise on the powerful potential of learning from mistakes.

Clinical risk management is not only about acting on mistakes to prevent them re-occurring. It is also about the prevention of errors through training of all members of the PHCT and the development and implementation of policies to promote safe practices. Sometimes an error is detected or intercepted early before it has had the opportunity to cause harm. Such 'near misses' need to be acknowledged – not ignored or brushed under the carpet. Ignoring or forgetting about these near misses may increase the likelihood of them being repeated at another time when they may not be intercepted before causing harm.

Staff and organisational development

The success of clinical governance will largely depend on staff and organisational development, the importance of which was described in Chapter 5. Without addressing the environment and the culture in which healthcare is delivered, it is unlikely that the quality of healthcare will improve. This will involve paying attention to the:

- physical environment
- administrative environment
- learning environment.

The physical environment

This refers to the conditions in which healthcare staff work and learn. Delivery of high quality healthcare cannot be expected without good working conditions and adequate resources. At a basic level, the environment should have warmth, light, ventilation, cleanliness and space. It needs to be welcoming for patients and healthcare staff.

The administrative environment

This refers to the systems and processes that enable us to perform our work. It entails having clear and achievable guidelines regarding registering patients, taking messages, making appointments, dealing with urgent requests. It would also cover the processes of communication between the practice and its patients as well as between the individual members of the primary healthcare team. It needs to be supported by good clinical and administrative equipment (telephone, fax machines, computers, medical records and so on).

The learning environment

This refers to fostering further learning and development and was considered in Chapter 5. It concerns psychosocial factors, such as breaking of social barriers and building a culture of openness, respect, trust and honesty within a democratic organisation. It encompasses how the individual members of the PHCT relate to each other and the value placed on individual and collaborative learning.

PCGs have the freedom to develop their own priorities and their own methods for facilitating and monitoring clinical governance based upon local issues and needs. They will be accountable for ensuring clinical governance takes place within each of their practices. Practices will also be accountable and will have appointed a clinical governance lead. He or she will co-ordinate the process of clinical governance and be able to produce evidence that it is taking place. The toolbox aims to provide a mechanism to demonstrate that clinical governance is taking place. In Part Three, Section D, examples are provided for each of the 'five pillars' of clinical governance and addressing these areas will successfully address the needs of clinical governance.

Part Two

Your personal and practice profile

Personal profile

Include a copy of your job description and contract and any other information you feel relevant. You may wish to use your CV, if you have one, for this section. If not, complete the following:

Date: . . . .

Part 1

Personal details	
Name	
Address Tel Fax Email	
Date of birth	
Qualifications/awards (dates and awarding body)	
Present position held and date appointed (include time devoted)	

Any other current appointments (include time devoted)	
List any interests or specific responsibilities within the practice (clinical or non-clinical)	
List previous relevant job experience	

Part 2

Registration details	
GMC/UKCC registration number	
Type of registration	
Date specialist registration was obtained	
Date of last revalidation	
Describe and date any breaks in your registration during the revalidation period	
Describe and date any conditions that have been placed on your registration	
Describe and date any erasure or suspension of registration imposed on you	

Part 3

Teaching, research and publications	
Teaching experience/ presentations	
Research	

Publications	

Practice profile

Date: . . . .

Practice area	
Urban/rural	
Particular geographical, social and environmental features (e.g. social mix, social features, employment levels, local issues, disease preponderance)	

Premises	
Building	Owned ☐ Rented ☐ Purpose built ☐ Converted ☐
Consulting rooms	No ☐
Treatment rooms	No ☐
Common rooms	No ☐
Ancillary staff rooms	No ☐
Other rooms (e.g. library, study, seminar, please specify)	
Describe how the practice building caters for the disabled person (i.e. wheelchair access, disabled toilet etc.)	
Other specific features of the premises	

Primary healthcare team (PHCT)		
	No	*Full-time/part-time (hours/week)*
Doctor(s)		
Nurse(s)		
Practice manager		
Secretary		
Receptionists		
Health visitor		
District nurse		
Midwife		
Dietician		
Counsellor		
Others		

Practice meetings	
	How often?
PHCT	
Staff	
Management	
Audit	
Educational	
Other	

Patient population profile							
Current list size							
Age	0–4	5–15	16–44	44–64	65–74	75–84	84+
Male							
Female							
Totals							

How does your list size compare to last year? List any reasons for change.

Practice features	
Appointment system	Yes ☐ No ☐
Medical records	Records in chronological order? Yes ☐ No ☐ Records summarised?　　　　　　Yes ☐ No ☐
Computer	System: Is the computer used for: ☐ repeat prescribing　　☐ acute prescribing ☐ limited disease index　☐ full disease index ☐ targets　☐ audits　　☐ appointments ☐ record of consultation　☐ consultation details
Internet access	Yes ☐　　No ☐
Library	Yes ☐　　No ☐
Special diagnostic equipment	
Teaching	Postgraduate ☐　　Undergraduate ☐　　Other ☐

Practice work		
Clinics held	*How often?*	*Protocols*
Antenatal		Yes ☐ No ☐
Asthma		Yes ☐ No ☐
Child health		Yes ☐ No ☐
Diabetes		Yes ☐ No ☐
Elderly		Yes ☐ No ☐
Family planning		Yes ☐ No ☐
Hypertension/heart disease		Yes ☐ No ☐
Travel		Yes ☐ No ☐
Minor surgery		Yes ☐ No ☐
Other		Yes ☐ No ☐

Targets							
Childhood immunisation 2y	*Dip Tet Pol*	*Pert*	*MMR*	*HIB*	*Childhood immunisation 5y*		*Pre-school booster*
90%							
70%							
Cervical cytology					*Comments*		
80%							
50%							

Patients' voice	
How do the patients contribute towards the practice development (e.g. suggestion box, questionnaires, patients' association)	

Specific innovations	
Are there any special features of your practice you wish to mention?	

Part Three

The learning activity templates

How to use the templates

The Toolbox for Portfolio Development is for all members of the PHCT, i.e. receptionists, practice managers, nurses, PAMs and doctors. Members of the team should have their own copy but the practice may wish to develop a portfolio for the practice as a whole. This may be particularly useful for tackling the area of clinical governance.

Part Three contains all the learning activity templates. It is divided into four sections.

    Section A: Learning from patients.
    Section B: Learning from colleagues.
    Section C: Learning from our personal experiences and life events.
    Section D: Addressing clinical governance.

The first two sections contain examples of learning activity templates. Some you may find useful and suited to your style of learning and you may wish to work through these templates. Alternatively, you may wish to modify or adapt them. It is probably easiest if you keep a single portfolio for each year. Although you cannot hope to complete all the templates, try and provide a handful of examples from each section.

Section D addresses how you will be able to use the learning activity templates to provide evidence of clinical governance. This section is subdivided into five areas:

- audit
- clinical effectiveness
- clinical risk management

- quality assurance
- staff and organisational development.

To show that you are addressing clinical governance issues, you will need to provide examples from each of these areas.

Section A: Learning from patients

Overview of learning activity templates

Template	Overview
For all members of the PHCT	
A1	Identifying individual strengths/weaknesses
A2	Personal education plan
A3	Patient interaction logs: identifying needs
A4	Significant event analysis
A5	Learning from complaints
A6	Learning from mistakes or near misses
A7	Learning from positives
A8	Learning from audits

For clinical members	
A9	Identifying individual strengths/weaknesses
A10	Personal education plan
A11	Consultation analysis – self-assessment
A12	Consultation analysis – self-assessment
A13	Consultation analysis – patient assessment (PEI)
A14	Consultation analysis – patient assessment (DISQ)
A15	Learning from PACT data

A1 and A2 Identifying individual strengths and weaknesses (self-appraisal for non-clinical topics) and a personal education plan

You can carry out this exercise on your own or, in order to obtain a more objective appraisal, you may find it useful to carry it out with another member of the primary healthcare team.

This exercise is a variation on the SWOT analysis. SWOT is an acronym for Strengths, Weaknesses, Opportunities and Threats. Any organisation will have strengths and weakness as well as opportunities the practice can capitalise on and threats that might impede progress or change. It can be used as a framework for beginning to examine improvements within the practice with the purpose of introducing change which hopefully will lead to improvement in the quality of care. The exercise can be carried out by an individual or a group, each area being tackled in turn. At the end of the exercise, it is possible to draw upon a list of issues that need to be addressed.

You may choose to look at your individual or your PHCT's strengths and weaknesses only in an area of healthcare. The templates in Section A deal with self-appraisal for non-clinical topics (A1 and A2) or clinical topics (A9 and A10). The PHCT as a whole can carry out a similar exercise (*see* Section B – B1 and B2 where an example is also provided). There are two templates to complete: the first identifies your strengths and weaknesses in a given area; the second allows you to complete an education action plan.

Step 1: *Identify your strengths and weaknesses* (A1) in each of the listed areas, i.e. what are you doing well and how can you do better? Complete the appropriate row for each category if relevant.

Step 2: Having identified your gaps and your learning needs, *complete your personal education plan* (A2) for this subject. There are two sections to the personal education plan. The first section concerns planning and managing your learning:

- identifying what you need to know
- how you will approach the subject

- what help or support you will need
- what the learning outcomes will look like.

The second section concerns evaluating your plan after you have embarked on the learning:

- did you achieve your goals?
- the conclusions or changes that resulted
- any new learning need identified.

A1 Identifying individual strengths/weaknesses

Date: . . . .

	Identify individual strengths (What am I doing well?)	Identify individual weaknesses (What can I do better?)
Interface with patients (e.g. ability to communicate, attitude to patients, ability to handle difficult patients, recognising seriously ill patients, dealing with emergencies)		
Teamwork (e.g. working as a member of a team, relationship with other members, communication with other members of the team)		
Knowledge of work (knowing and understanding aspects of work relevant to job)		

Skills and task-related work (e.g. telephone skills, computer skills, procedural skills, organisational skills, clear written records)		
Attitude to work (time management, willingness, sickness record, motivation and commitment, ability to work under pressure)		
Professional issues (ability to use initiative, attitude to continuing development, ability to self appraise performance, ability to change, ability to accept and use constructive criticism, assertiveness skills)		

A2 Personal education plan

Planning and managing learning
What do I/we need to learn? What questions are to be answered?
What are the outcomes or benefits?
How will I/we do it? What resources are needed? Time required?
How will I/we show what I/we have learnt? What will the outcome look like?
How will I and my practice and, crucially, the patients benefit?

Evaluating learning
Were the learning goals achieved? If not, why not?
What conclusions or changes have resulted?
Are there any other learning needs that have been discovered?
Signed by learner: . . . .   Signed by mentor: . . . .   Date: . . . .

A3 Patient interaction logs: identifying needs

You cannot be expected to know the answers to everything but you must be prepared and honest enough to admit when you do not know.

Having identified your learning need, you must also be prepared to correct your deficiency and attempt to find the answer. Scribbling the question or the learning need on a piece of paper is not often successful. If you do find the paper, several weeks later, the urgency, immediacy, and the meaning or relevance of the problem have vanished.

This template allows you to systematically record any questions or needs that arise during interaction with patients. It is important not only to record the problem and the learning needs question but also how you will go about finding the answer. The last column allows you to record the outcome of your learning.

A3 Patient interaction logs: identifying needs

Record any consultations or interactions with patients where a question has arisen – where you have identified a learning need. This may be a knowledge gap or improving or acquiring a new skill. State how you plan to address this need and complete the outcome column.

Week beginning: . . . .

Patient ID No.	Problem	Learning needs question	Action How will you find the answer?	Outcome? Comments

A4 Significant event analysis

Significant events or critical incident exercises[10,25,26] have been used for many years in continuing professional development and are a valuable learning tool. The significant event technique prompts you to identify an incident that for some reason was of particular significance to you. It could be anything from an unexplained death, communication difficulties (with patients or colleagues), an aggressive or difficult patient, a complaint, a drug side effect, or a prescribing or procedural error. It may be any incident or event that has been different to the usual 'routine' and it might have left you feeling happy or frustrated. Because these events have stuck in your mind and are often charged with emotion, they are particularly useful learning situations. Try and write a short description or summary about an event that occurs during the course of your work. Reflecting upon the event and your summary may help to clarify some unresolved issues. This will help you to make some interpretations and help you identify learning outcomes.

Ideally the event is best shared with a colleague(s) (i.e. pairs, triads, a large group or the practice team). This should help the process of critical reflection and maximise the learning. It is important that the culture is 'right'. There must be honesty, trust and respect within the team.

Using the structured approach described in this template may help you make the most of the event and a more meaningful outcome may be achieved. You could begin by attempting the exercise below.[20]

Exercise:

Think back over the past 6–12 months. During that time, was there an incident that made you feel, as a health professional, a real high of excitement, satisfaction or fulfilment? A time when you said to yourself, 'This is what makes my job worthwhile'? Write a brief description of the event on a sheet of A4.

Now repeat the exercise with an incident that caused you concern, despair or a sense of failure. It might have been an event that made you feel awful, humiliated. A time when you said to yourself, 'I am not enjoying being in this job'. Write a brief description of the event on a sheet of A4.

A4 Significant event analysis: a structured approach

Date: . . . .

Describe what happened: What did you do and what actually happened?

Describe your feelings: What were you thinking or feeling at the time? What were the consequences for (a) the patient, (b) others, (c) yourself and what were they feeling?

Make a judgement: What were you trying to achieve and what was good or bad about it?

Analyse: What factors were influencing you? What knowledge or skills would have helped you?

Draw a conclusion: What can you conclude from this experience? How does it relate to your previous experiences? Faced with this experience again, what would you do?

Make an action learning plan: What are you going to do differently next time and how will you address any learning needs?

A5 and A6 Learning from negatives: complaints, mistakes or near misses

In recent years, the number of complaints against health staff has been gradually rising. Although distressing to the patient and the practice, complaints or mistakes need not necessarily be seen in a negative light. It needs to be acknowledged that mistakes can and do occur. Mistakes are an essential part of learning and everybody makes them. They should not be allowed to undermine self-esteem.

Mistakes are a mechanism by which you can strive to improve the quality of care you provide. You may strive to avoid mistakes but in reality they do happen and 'to err is human'. That does not mean they can be dismissed. It is important to try and look at complaints in a positive way. In the same way as audit, they can be a mechanism for identifying deficiencies in the service you provide. It is important to avoid being secretive and defensive and to provide time to reflect upon any mistakes or complaints and to examine any learning outcomes.

Near misses can also be educational. A near miss today may become a serious mistake and a complaint tomorrow. Lessons need to be learnt from near misses to avoid this.

A5 and A6 will help provide opportunities for learning from complaints, mistakes or near misses.

A5 Learning from complaints

Date: . . . .

Review any complaints you have received in the last three months
List the major points regarding the complaint
How was this complaint resolved?
What if anything have you or the practice learnt from the complaint?
What action has been planned or taken as a result of this learning?

A6 Learning from mistakes or near misses

Date: . . . .

Review any mistakes or near misses that you have observed or have been pointed out to you
List the major points regarding the mistake or near miss
How did it occur? What reasons might explain its occurrence?
What if anything have you or the practice learnt from the mistake or near miss?
What action has been planned or taken as a result of this learning?

A7 Learning from positives

Focusing on mistakes and your learning needs can be a little disconcerting and de-motivating and undermine your self-esteem. Occasionally it is necessary to build yourself up and acknowledge some of your positive attributes. By acknowledging the positives and celebrating what you do well, you will not only improve your self-confidence but you will also learn a great deal from analysing your strengths.

You may be naturally modest or disinclined to provide evidence of things you do well. But, just as you can learn from mistakes, so you can also learn from praise. Sometimes you may do things well and not be aware of them, as they do not appear obvious to you or you may take them for granted. By recognising your strengths and the things you do well, you will be able to build upon them.

Include in this section anything that will demonstrate things you do well. This may include your own assessment or those of others, comments from colleagues or grateful letters from patients. You may wish to see if you can draw any observations or further learning from the praise received.

A8 Learning from audits

Audit has become an acceptable part of general practice. If the quality of healthcare is to improve, then regular auditing of care must be undertaken. Audit concerns the systematic process of critically analysing the quality of healthcare through measurement and evaluation. Its objective is to improve the quality of care provided through the introduction of change and monitoring the effects of this change. Certain key steps characterise the process and a successful audit is one that addresses all the steps (*see* Chapter 7).

Audits should not be carried out for auditing's sake. You need to be quite clear why you are undertaking the audit and you need to ensure that the audit covers a wide area of healthcare delivery.

This learning activity template is divided into four sections covering audits in acute care, chronic care, practice management, and screening and prevention. List the audits that you or the practice has undertaken and, for each one, try to provide the following:

- a description of the audit, the standards used and how they were decided upon
- why this particular area was chosen
- the change or outcome resulting from the audit to the service or patient care
- who was involved in the audit, i.e. was it doctors, all clinical staff, or administrative staff as well
- whether the audit cycle has been repeated.

Most practices are familiar with carrying out audits in chronic conditions such as asthma, diabetes or hypertension. However, audits should also be carried out in other areas of healthcare, the way the practice is run, or whether screening programmes are undertaken effectively. Audits, therefore, may be seen to cover the following areas:

- acute care
- chronic care
- practice management
- screening and prevention.

It is important to provide a range of audits and for this reason, A8 provides the templates to cover the above areas.

A8 Learning from audits

Provide a summary of how you have addressed this area on this page and include examples/evidence of any of the following in your portfolio:

Audits in acute care

Date	Brief description of audit including standards	Why was this audit selected?	Change or outcome resulting from audit	Who was involved in the audit?	Audit cycle repeated?

Audits in chronic care

Date	Brief description of audit including standards	Why was this audit selected?	Change or outcome resulting from audit	Who was involved in the audit?	Audit cycle repeated?

Audits in practice management

Date	Brief description of audit including standards	Why was this audit selected?	Change or outcome resulting from audit	Who was involved in the audit?	Audit cycle repeated?

Audits in screening and prevention

Date	Brief description of audit including standards	Why was this audit selected?	Change or outcome resulting from audit	Who was involved in the audit?	Audit cycle repeated?

A9 and A10 Identifying individual strengths and weaknesses (self-appraisal for clinical topics) and a personal education plan

This exercise is similar to A1 and A2 but is more suited for clinical areas.

You can carry out this exercise on your own or, in order to obtain a more objective appraisal, you may find it useful to carry it out with another member of the primary healthcare team.

It is a variation on the SWOT analysis. SWOT is an acronym for **S**trengths, **W**eaknesses, **O**pportunities and **T**hreats. Any organisation will have strengths and weakness as well as opportunities the practice can capitalise on and threats that might impede progress or change. It can be used as a framework for beginning to examine improvements within the practice with the purpose of introducing change which will hopefully lead to improvement in the quality of care. The exercise can be carried out by an individual or a group, each area being tackled in turn. At the end of the exercise, it is possible to draw upon a list of issues that need to be addressed.

You may choose to look at your individual or your primary healthcare team's strengths and weaknesses only in an area of healthcare. These templates deal with self-appraisal for clinical topics. The primary healthcare team as a whole can carry out a similar exercise (*see* Section B – B1 and B2 where an example is also provided). There are two templates to complete: the first identifies your strengths and weaknesses in a given area; the second allows you to complete an education action plan.

Step 1: Identify a clinical area that you wish to focus on. It may be a perceived need or a subject of current interest, or have been identified for you as a need that should be addressed. If possible obtain an objective view of your needs through the help of a mentor.

Step 2: *Identify your strengths* in each of the listed areas, i.e. what are *you* doing well? Complete the appropriate row for each category if relevant.

Step 3: *Identify your weaknesses* in each of the listed areas, i.e. how can *you* do better? Complete the appropriate row for each category if relevant.

Step 4: If possible discuss with your mentor. Alternatively reflect on your analysis on your own.

Step 5: Having identified your gaps and your learning needs, *complete your personal education plan* (A10) for this subject. There are two sections to the personal education plan. The first section concerns planning and managing your learning:

- identifying what you need to know
- how you will approach the subject
- what help or support you will need
- what the learning outcomes will look like.

Step 6: The second section concerns evaluating your plan after you have embarked on the learning:

- did you achieve your goals?
- the conclusions or changes that resulted
- any new learning need identified.

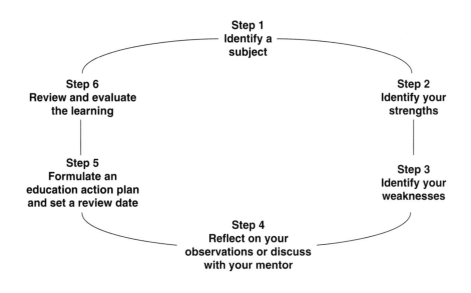

Identifying learning needs: strengths/weaknesses

A9 Identifying individual strengths/weaknesses

Date: . . . .   Subject: . . . .

	Identify individual strengths (What am I doing well?)	*Identify individual weaknesses (What can I do better?)*
Acute care		
Chronic care		
Screening or preventive care		

	Identify individual strengths (What am I doing well?)	*Identify individual weaknesses (What can I do better?)*
Practical skills		
Management		
Audit		

A10 Personal education plan

Date: . . . .   Subject: . . . .

Planning and managing learning
What do I need to learn? What questions are to be answered?
What are the outcomes or benefits?
How will I do it? What resources are needed? Time required?
How will I show what I have learnt? What will the outcome look like?
How will I and my practice and, crucially, the patients benefit?

Evaluating learning
Were the learning goals achieved? If not, why not?
What conclusions or changes have resulted?
Are there any other learning needs that have been discovered?
Signed by learner: . . . .   Signed by mentor: . . . . Date: . . . .

A11 and A12 Consultation analysis: self-assessment

Analysing consultations can be a valuable and useful method of improving the way you interact and relate with patients. You can do this on your own but ideally you should recruit the help of a colleague or colleagues. There are four templates that are included here. The first two are concerned with a self-assessment of your consultation. These assessments may be carried out retrospectively after your consultation. However, more useful information and learning can be obtained by the use of a video. This is then observed after the consultation, with a colleague or within a group. The feedback received can help provide you with an appraisal of your consultation skills.

A11 Consultation analysis: self-assessment

Date: . . . .

Good and difficult consultations
Which was the most satisfying or successful consultation in the last week? Why do you think it was successful?
Which was the most difficult problem consultation you have had in the last week? Why was it difficult? What would you do differently next time?

A12 Consultation analysis: self-assessment

Date: . . . .

What do you think was the patients' reason for attendance?

Were you able to identify this?

Do you think you responded appropriately:

* non-verbally?
* verbally?

What were you able to achieve? What did you do well?

What were you not able to achieve? How could you have done better?

What have you learnt and what do you need to change?

What is your action plan now? How will you improve?

A13 and A14 Consultation analysis: patient assessment

These two questionnaires provide an analysis of patients' assessment of their consultation with you.

The *patient enablement instrument* (PEI) has been developed by the Department of General Practice in Edinburgh.[27] It aims to provide an outcome measure of primary care consultations. Enablement is seen as related, but different, to satisfaction. The emphasis is on patient-centredness and empowerment and the ability of patients to understand and cope with their health and illness. Patients may be asked to complete the questionnaire following the consultation. The PEI consists of six questions only, making it simple to use and score. Scoring of the PEI is as follows:

'same' or 'less' (response in right-hand column) – score 0
'better' or 'more' (response in middle column) – score 1
'much better' or 'much more' (response in left-hand column) – score 2.

The possible range of scores is from zero (respondent answered 'same' or 'less' to all six questions) to a maximum of 12 (respondent answered 'much better' or 'much more' to all six questions).

The *doctors' interpersonal skills questionnaire* (DISQ) has been developed by the Royal Australian College of General Practitioners to provide feedback to GP registrars and other GPs on their interpersonal skills within the consultation.[28] DISQ consists of 12 questions for patients to complete at the end of each consultation. There is a five-point evaluation scale from 'excellent' to 'poor'.

A13 Patient enablement instrument

Date: . . . .

Please tick appropriate box.

	Much better	Better	Same or less	Not applicable
As a result of your visit to the doctor today, do you feel you are:				
• able to cope with life				
• able to understand your illness				
• able to cope with your illness				
• able to keep yourself healthy				
• confident about your health				
• able to help yourself				

A14 Doctors' interpersonal skills questionnaire (DISQ)

Date: . . . .

Please score (tick) the following statements after your visit with the doctor.

		Excellent	Very good	Good	Fair	Poor
1	My overall satisfaction with the visit to the doctor is . . .					
2	The warmth of the doctor's greeting to me was . . .					
3	On this visit, I would rate the doctor's ability to listen to me as . . .					
4	The doctor's explanations of things to me were . . .					
5	The extent to which I felt reassured by this doctor was . . .					
6	My confidence in this doctor's ability is . . .					
7	The opportunity the doctor gave me to express my concerns or fears was . . .					
8	The respect shown to me by this doctor was . . .					
9	The time given to me for this visit was . . .					
10	The doctor's consideration in deciding a treatment for me was . . .					
11	The doctor's concern for me as a person in this visit was . . .					
12	The recommendation I would give to my friends about this doctor would be . . .					

A15 Learning from PACT data

The Prescription Pricing Authority (PPA) produces prescribing analysis and cost (PACT) data – a quarterly report analysing the prescribing costs of individual doctors and their practice. Looking at prescribing patterns can be a valuable way of looking at issues of quality and the PACT data provide a mechanism for doing this. The PACT standard report contains prescribing costs compared with local HA and national patterns. It presents some data as prescribing units; patients under 65 count as one prescribing unit and those over 65 as three prescribing units (PUs).

Through an examination of the PACT data sent to you, you should be able to audit your own prescribing habits. The report presents trends in prescribing throughout the country on a specific topic and also presents your individual prescribing patterns on the drugs under review. The centre blue pages provide a useful educational input on important prescribing issues. A fuller prescribing catalogue is available on request, which can be used for a more specific and detailed analysis of prescribing, for example the use of specific drugs and their generic prescribing rates.

PACT data can be difficult to interpret. This template offers an opportunity to look at the costs of prescribing, the 20 leading drugs and your generic prescribing. You may wish to include your PACT report and an analysis of it in your portfolio.

A15 Learning from PACT data

Quarter ending: . . . .

Practice prescribing costs			
	Amount	*Change from last year (%)*	*% above (+) or below (−) HA*
Your practice			
HA equivalent			
Your own costs			

- If there are differences between your individual/practice prescribing costs and the HA equivalent, can you think of any reasons for this?

- Has there been any significant change from last year? If so, what are the reasons for this?

Your practice costs by BNF group

- If there are differences between your practice prescribing costs by BNF therapeutic group and the HA equivalent, can you think of any reasons for this?

- Has there been any significant change from last year? If so, what are the reasons for this?

The 20 leading cost drugs in your practice

- Look at this group. Information is provided regarding (a) total costs, (b) % of practice total, (c) % change from last year and (d) number of items. What observations can you make from these figures? Is any action required by the practice?

The number of items prescribed generically was: . . . .

- Is this an area the practice can improve upon? If so, how?

Conclusions and action plan

- Draw some final conclusions on the PACT data.

- Make an action plan to deal with any recommendations.

Section B: Learning from colleagues

Overview of learning activity templates

Template	Overview
For all members of the PHCT	
B1	Identifying practice strengths and weaknesses
B2	Practice education plan
B3	Learning from outside events
B4	Inter-professional learning
B5	In-house education events
B6	Learning with other practices
B7	Self-appraisal form
B8	Appraisal from others
B9	Appraisal form: skills related
B10	Development of guidelines or protocols
B11	Learning from external guidelines (National Service Frameworks)
B12	Learning from risk management
B13	Critical reading

For clinical members	
B14	Critical reading: scientific/clinical articles
B15	Consultation analysis: video analysis

B1 and B2 Identifying practice strengths and weaknesses and a practice education plan

This exercise is a variation on the SWOT analysis. SWOT is an acronym for Strengths, Weaknesses, Opportunities and Threats. Any organisation will have strengths and weakness as well as opportunities the practice can capitalise on and threats that might impede progress or change. It can be used as a framework for beginning to examine improvements within the practice with the purpose of introducing change which will hopefully lead to improvement in the quality of care. The exercise can be carried out by an individual or a group, each area being tackled in turn. At the end of the exercise, it is possible to draw upon a list of issues that need to be addressed.

You may wish to carry out a SWOT exercise or alternatively these templates deal with strengths and weaknesses. They aim to discover your primary healthcare team's strengths and weaknesses in an area of healthcare. There are two templates to complete: the first identifies your team's strengths and weaknesses in a given area; the second allows the team to complete a practice education plan.

Step 1: The primary healthcare team (PHCT) should meet and *identify a subject* they wish to focus on in greater depth. To identify the subject, it may be necessary to brainstorm. It may be a perceived need that may have been identified or it may be a subject of interest or importance to the practice.

Step 2: In B1, the PHCT should try and identify *the practice's strengths* in this area, i.e. what are *we* doing well? Complete the appropriate row for each category if relevant.

Step 3: Now do the same for areas of weakness. In B1, identify *the practice's weaknesses* in this area, i.e. how can *we* do better? Complete the appropriate row for each category if relevant.

Step 4: The PHCT should then meet and discuss the results of the two templates regarding strengths and weaknesses. Share each other's ideas, in a group or in subgroups, regarding the strengths of the practice. It is important to recognise what the practice is doing well, to acknowledge it and to celebrate it. Now focus on the areas of weakness in the practice. How can things be improved?

Step 5: At the end of the discussion try and identify a *practice education plan* (B2) to deal with the areas of weakness and further learning needs. It may be that changes will need to be made as to how the practice is organised and this will involve the whole PHCT. On the other hand, individuals may have discovered a learning need that they need to be addressed and they will need to form their own action plan.

Step 6: At the conclusion of the plan, evaluate the learning.

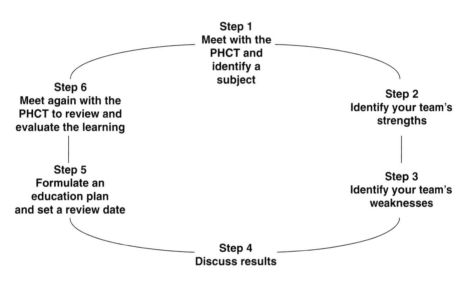

Identifying learning needs: strengths/weaknesses

For example, if your team has chosen diabetes, your template might look like this:

	Strengths	*Weaknesses*
Acute care	• We are able to provide urgent appointments • We are aware of the symptoms of the acute presentation of a newly diagnosed diabetic	• Receptionists not aware of symptoms of hypos • Need to provide a hotline for diabetics to contact us easily
Chronic care	• We run an effective diabetic clinic and provide annual assessment of feet, eyes and kidney as well as focusing on hyperlipidaemia, BP and diabetes control	• Treatment threshold for raised cholesterol could be lower • BP control needs improvement in many diabetics • Many diabetics, control is poor • Probably could do more to get diabetics to stop smoking
Screening/ preventive care	• All new patients screened for diabetes	• We need to screen high-risk groups more efficiently
Practical skills	• We provide fundoscopy	• Skills for detecting retinopathy need improvement
Management	• Our recall system works well • Our disease template is well constructed	• We sometimes miss our defaulters • Housebound diabetics get less attention – less monitoring
Audit	• We run an annual audit	• We do not always act on the results of the audit

With a long list of weaknesses, it is easy to get demoralised and de-motivated but focusing initially on one or two weaknesses and delegating tasks to individual members of the team may help. For example, the doctor responsible for fundoscopy may decide to further his skills in this area by attending a course. The practice manager could look at the need for a hotline. The receptionist might be provided with information on hypos and the nurses may look at the development of a protocol for screening.

A practice education plan will need to be completed, as well as personal education plans. The practice will then need to meet after a timeframe has been decided.

B1 Identifying practice strengths/weaknesses

Date: . . . .   The subject is: . . . .

	Identify practice strengths (What are we doing well?)	*Identify practice weaknesses (How can we do better?)*
Acute care		
Chronic care		
Screening / preventive care		

	Identify practice strengths (What are we doing well?)	*Identify practice weaknesses (How can we do better?)*
Practical skills		
Management		
Audit		

B2 Practice education plan

Date: . . . .   The subject is: . . . .

Planning and managing learning
What do we need to learn/change? What questions are to be answered? What needs to be done?
What are the outcomes or benefits?
How will we do it? What resources are needed? Time required?
How will we show what we have learnt/changed? What will the outcome look like?
How will the practice and, crucially, the patients benefit?

Evaluating learning
Were the outcomes achieved? If not, why not?
What conclusions or changes have resulted?
Are there any other learning needs that have been discovered or any further changes needed?
Signed on behalf of PHCT: . . . . Date: . . . .

B3 Learning from outside events

Learning from courses, meetings or lectures is a time-honoured method for most in primary care. It is preferred by many. There is a danger that attending lectures encourages passivity. To avoid this and to make sure that you make the most of the learning situation, you need to take control of your learning from outside events. It is not sufficient just to list any courses, meetings and lectures that you have attended.

Before you attend any meeting, course or lecture, try to identify what you hope to gain by attending. Why are you attending? Following the event, identify what the main learning points or outcomes have been and how they may be applicable to your work.

B3 Learning from outside events

Review before the event	
Date/venue	
Course/lecture title	
What do I hope to learn/achieve?	

First review after the event	
Was this learning achieved?	
How will you be able to apply your new learning to your work?	
Set a second review date for evaluating the learning	

Second review after the event	
Date of review	
Have you been able to apply your new learning?	
What have been the benefits to patients, the practice, yourself?	

B4 Inter-professional learning

To provide successful and integrated healthcare to your patients, you need to work with other professions in a team approach. There are a large number of professions that are involved in the provision of healthcare. These may be the more obvious members of the PHCT, i.e. doctors, nurses, health visitors, administrative staff and so on. Other health professionals may not be such obvious members of the PHCT. These may include occupational therapists, physiotherapists or complementary therapists. Each has their own perspective on healthcare. But despite the differences, you share a common denominator, which places the client or patient at the foreground. There is much to be gained from understanding how different healthcare professions work and how they can function effectively as a team. Sometimes an insight can develop; a view from a different perspective, or a flash of understanding. Unless this can be recorded, it may be lost.

You may wish to list examples of any opportunities you have had of learning with and from other health professionals. The list of 'other health professionals' is broad and may include not only members of the PHCT but also complementary therapists, pharmacists, speech therapists and any PAM. Try to identify what it is you learnt and if you will be able to apply it to your practice. Have there been any changes of attitudes as a result?

B4 Inter-professional learning

Event	Professions represented	Learning outcome	Application to practice

B5 In-house education events
B6 Learning with other practices

Many practices now provide for their own education and continuing development. These may or may not involve other health professionals or outside speakers. Formal meetings may concern audit, prescribing, new knowledge, refining clinical skills, for example resuscitation, or practice management. You can provide a log of these in B5.

Some practices have joined together for the purposes of sharing their education and continuing development. This may take the form of a shared audit, a presentation, critical reading, improving computer skills or comparison/development of shared guidelines. Providing a log of these and completing B6 will help demonstrate evidence of learning.

B5 In-house education events

Date	Subject	Who was present	Learning method	Main learning outcomes	Action plan

B6 Learning with other practices

Date	Subject	Who was present	Learning method	Main learning outcomes	Action plan

B7, B8 and B9 Appraisals

Effective healthcare delivery is dependent on an efficient PHCT. Each member of the primary healthcare team needs to be quite clear about their role and their job description within the practice. Most people do want to know how they are performing in their work and will welcome an opportunity to be appraised. A system of regular appraisal is an opportunity to review the performance of a member of the team.

It is important to acknowledge that appraisal is a two-way process. The person being appraised must also engage in self-appraisal in addition to the appraiser offering his or her own assessment. It is a formative process designed not only to improve the performance of the individual but also to facilitate their professional development and help maximise their potential within the practice.

To achieve successful appraisal, a formal structured process must be observed. If an appraisal system does not already exist in the practice, then an opportunity should be provided for a general discussion concerning the structure and mechanism of the intended system, with all the members of the PHCT. It needs to be made explicit that the appraisal should be conducted upon the basis of mutual trust and respect. All members of the team including the doctors should be appraised. Who conducts the appraisal should also be discussed. Usually the practice manager, alone or with a GP, could appraise the administrative staff. The GPs could appraise the practice manager and the GPs (with or without the practice manager) could appraise the nurses and each other.

A formal letter of invitation should be sent together with a self-appraisal form. This form is completed by the person being appraised, who brings it to the interview. The appraiser completes a similar form about the person being appraised. These will form the basis of the discussion.

The *Oxford English Dictionary* defines appraise, as an '*estimate (of) the amount, quality, or excellence*'. At the end of the process, the person having been appraised should feel that they have been listened to and they should have a clear idea about:

- their strengths
- their weaknesses
- their achievements

- the standards expected
- the ways in which they could improve their performance
- how the practice could help them develop
- how to address their learning needs
- an action plan for the next 12 months.

B7 and B8 are similar, but B7 is an appraisal form that is completed by the person being appraised and the appraiser completes B8. Both are brought to the interview for discussion. B9 is much more task-orientated and again both the appraiser and the person being appraised should complete identical forms.

Example letter of invitation

Dear

I am pleased to offer you the following appointment for your annual appraisal of your performance in your work as a . . . . (job title) . . . . The appraisal will take place on . . . . at . . . . and will be conducted by . . . .

This will provide us with an opportunity to assess your strengths, the areas in which you can improve and how the practice can help you to take forward your professional development.

I enclose a self-appraisal form which you should complete and bring to your appointment. This will help us identify relevant areas for discussion. I will be using a similar form to complete an appraisal of you. I look forward to seeing you then.

B7 Self-appraisal form

Part 1: Review
At my last appraisal, the following needs were identified:
Which of the above did you achieve and how has it benefited you and your practice?
Which learning needs have you not been able to achieve? Please state why you were unable to achieve them.

Part 2: Current appraisal

What do I do well?

How does the practice/PHCT help me achieve this?

What or how could I do better?

List your most significant achievements in the last 12 months

Is there anything you would have liked to have achieved?

What prevented you from doing this?

What would you like to learn/develop/achieve in the next 12 months?			
What needs to be addressed?	*How will it be addressed?*	*Proposed outcome*	*Review date*

What could the practice do to help me achieve my goals?

What opportunities does the practice offer me (both now and for the future)?

What threats does the practice pose for me?

Is there anything else you want to talk about?

Signed (appraisee): . . . .   Signed (appraiser): . . . .

Date: . . . .

B8 Appraisal from others

What does he/she do well? How does the practice benefit?
List his/her most significant achievements in the last 12 months:
What or how could he/she do better?
What do you think prevented him/her from achieving this?
What could the practice or the team do to help him/her achieve his/her goals?
Was there anything else that was addressed at this appraisal?

Agreed action plan of learning needs identified:			
What needs to be addressed?	*How will it be addressed?*	*Proposed outcome*	*Review date*

Any other comments:

Signed (appraisee): . . . .   Signed (appraiser): . . . .

B9 Appraisal form: skills related

Before completing this form, read your job description. Complete the items in any sections that you feel apply to your role in the practice. Your appraiser will be completing an identical form. Both forms will need to be brought to the interview for discussion.

Name: . . . .   Date: . . . .

For each item indicate your rating by circling a number from 1 (poor) to 5 (very good).

	Applicable/ non-applicable	Rating	Comments
Interface with patients			
Presentation of self		1–2–3–4–5	
Communication skills		1–2–3–4–5	
Attitude to patients		1–2–3–4–5	
Ability to handle difficult patients		1–2–3–4–5	
Ability to recognise seriously ill patients		1–2–3–4–5	
Interpersonal relationship with individual patients		1–2–3–4–5	
Ability to implement the complaints procedure and deal with patient queries		1–2–3–4–5	
Establishes communication links with practice population		1–2–3–4–5	
Relationship to community		1–2–3–4–5	

	Applicable/ non-applicable	Rating	Comments
Ensures patient information systems are up to date		1–2–3–4–5	
Teamwork			
Works as a member of a team		1–2–3–4–5	
Relationship with administrative staff		1–2–3–4–5	
Relationship with clinical staff		1–2–3–4–5	
Communication with PHCT		1–2–3–4–5	
Contribution to PHCT development		1–2–3–4–5	
Contribution to meetings		1–2–3–4–5	
Management skills			
Time management skills		1–2–3–4–5	
Organisation of workload		1–2–3–4–5	
Ability to delegate and/or accept delegation		1–2–3–4–5	
Audits own performance		1–2–3–4–5	
Ability to accept change and implement change		1–2–3–4–5	
Assertiveness skills		1–2–3–4–5	

	Applicable/ non-applicable	*Rating*	*Comments*
Arranges practice meetings, agenda, minutes		1–2–3–4–5	
Organises protocols and ensures adherence		1–2–3–4–5	
Computer/record keeping			
Effective use of computer		1–2–3–4–5	
Ensures that computer system is running efficiently and securely		1–2–3–4–5	
Ensures regular computer back-ups		1–2–3–4–5	
Ability to run computer searches, audits, templates, recalls		1–2–3–4–5	
Maintains accurate records		1–2–3–4–5	
Ensures that medical records are in good order and filed		1–2–3–4–5	
Reception skills			
Telephone skills		1–2–3–4–5	
Making appointments		1–2–3–4–5	
Message taking		1–2–3–4–5	
Filing and other administrative tasks		1–2–3–4–5	

	Applicable/ non-applicable	Rating	Comments
Secretarial skills			
Ensures efficient handling of mail		1–2–3–4–5	
Maintains and updates accurate office filing system		1–2–3–4–5	
Minute taking skills		1–2–3–4–5	
Typing skills		1–2–3–4–5	
Ability to resolve patient queries		1–2–3–4–5	
Ability to liase with community trusts/ hospitals		1–2–3–4–5	
Keeps accurate log of referrals		1–2–3–4–5	
Ensures adequate stock levels		1–2–3–4–5	
Personnel management			
Organises rotas, cover for holidays and sickness		1–2–3–4–5	
Able to conduct effective staff appraisals		1–2–3–4–5	
Ensures appropriate training and continuing professional development		1–2–3–4–5	
Recruitment of staff		1–2–3–4–5	

	Applicable/ non-applicable	Rating	Comments
Prepares staff contracts, job descriptions		1–2–3–4–5	
Appropriately delegates tasks		1–2–3–4–5	
Liaises with staff and doctors to resolve problems		1–2–3–4–5	
Practice finances			
Runs an efficient petty cash system		1–2–3–4–5	
Pays bills and ensures money owed to practice is paid		1–2–3–4–5	
Keeps regular practice accounts		1–2–3–4–5	
Liases with bank and accountant		1–2–3–4–5	
Operates PAYE system, dealing with queries, end of year accounts, insurance and pensions		1–2–3–4–5	
Prepares budget and cash flow forecasts		1–2–3–4–5	
Ensures targets are achieved, organises recall systems and monitors IOS claims		1–2–3–4–5	
Records and submits all claim forms		1–2–3–4–5	

	Applicable/ non-applicable	Rating	Comments
Health centre management			
Ensures centre is well equipped, adequately stocked		1–2–3–4–5	
Maintains health and safety policy		1–2–3–4–5	
Makes policy decisions regarding efficient running of practice		1–2–3–4–5	
Deals with cleaning, maintenance and repairs		1–2–3–4–5	
Develops and maintains internal/external directories		1–2–3–4–5	
Deals with all practice publications and annual report		1–2–3–4–5	
Clinical work			
Range and application of clinical knowledge		1–2–3–4–5	
Range and application of clinical skills		1–2–3–4–5	
Adhering to protocols		1–2–3–4–5	
Prescribing skills		1–2–3–4–5	
Ability to deal with emergencies/resuscitation		1–2–3–4–5	
Interprets/responds to investigations		1–2–3–4–5	

	Applicable/ non-applicable	Rating	Comments
Referral of patients		1–2–3–4–5	
Personal and professional attitudes			
Motivation and commitment to work		1–2–3–4–5	
Ability to work under pressure		1–2–3–4–5	
Sickness record		1–2–3–4–5	
Ability to accept and use constructive criticism		1–2–3–4–5	
Ability to use initiative		1–2–3–4–5	
Commitment to continuing professional development		1–2–3–4–5	

- What are your/his/her strengths?

- What are your/his/her weaknesses?

- Please note here any specific points for discussion:

- Action plan for next 12 months (changes to be made in light of appraisal):

Signed (appraisee): . . . . Signed (appraiser): . . . . Date: . . . .

B10 Development of guidelines or protocols

Sometimes it is necessary to develop local or practice guidelines. It may be that none exist nationally or that the guidelines that do exist are not applicable. Alternatively the guidelines or protocol may refer to a system that needs to be personalised (e.g. a practice procedure such as repeat prescribing).

A great deal of learning can result from the research and negotiation involved in designing your own guideline. At the outset it is important to involve the whole team. It may be that a small subgroup is set up with the task of developing the guideline. Following its development, it will need to be disseminated to other members of the PHCT and its implementation and its success subjected to a review.

This template guides you through the process of the development of a guideline and providing documentary evidence of the process.

B10 Development of guidelines or protocols

Date: . . . .

What guideline is being developed?
Who was involved in its development?
What evidence/resources were used to support its development?

How has the guideline been disseminated?

Has the guideline been reviewed?

Changes resulting from review:

B11 Learning from external guidelines (National Service Frameworks)

Guidelines or standards may emerge from PCGs, HAs, NHSE regional offices or the national bodies such as the NSFs. Practices will be required to respond to them, make the necessary changes and be able to demonstrate that they are being addressed. This will require a team approach involving all members of the PHCT.

1 Identify the standard from the documents received.

2 It is better to start from your strengths and identify what you already do well in relation to this standard. Otherwise the team may feel de-motivated.

3 Having identified what you do well, identify what you need to do to achieve this standard. List the action points.

4 How will you do this? Which members of the team will be involved and what sorts of help or resources will you require?

5 Put a timescale on achieving and reviewing your progress.

6 Finally, indicate how you will be able to demonstrate your achievement. This could be entered into your portfolio on completion.

B11 Learning from external guidelines

Date: . . . .

List the standard:

What do we already do well in relation to this standard?

What do we need to do better to achieve this standard?
List the action points:

How will we do it? What resources will we need?

What is our timescale?

How will we be able to demonstrate our achievement?

B12 Learning from risk management

Risk management concerns reducing or eliminating the potential risk of harm to patients and staff in healthcare organisations. It is one of the 'pillars' of clinical governance. Successful risk management is about predicting the likely areas where risks might arise and developing strategies to ensure that they are avoided or minimised. It requires a team approach and this template will help you successfully address the potential risks in your practice.

It requires you to begin by identifying a subject for consideration. The subject may have been chosen because it has been recognised as one in which an error may occur or one in which the error may already have occurred. Subjects where risks might be identified come from the following areas:

- clinical conditions, e.g. acute, emergency or chronic care of any number of conditions
- clinical tasks or procedures, e.g. prescribing, treatment room, resuscitation etc.
- administrative, e.g. appointment system, medical records, computers etc.
- health and safety, e.g. aggressive patients, fire policy, first aid etc.
- ethical, e.g. confidentiality, disclosure of information etc.

B12 Learning from risk management

Date: . . . .

What is the subject?

Why was it chosen?

What are the potential risks?

How can the likelihood of these risks be avoided or minimised?

List the action points:

Has a guideline been developed? If so, include.

B13 Critical reading

Reading is essential to improve knowledge. Unless reading is approached in a systematic way, important information gained may not be retained. Browsing tends to be a superficial form of reading, where the reader tends to be passive and not relate in any involved way with the reading material. Browsing may not result in retention of relevant or significant information.

Critical reading, on the other hand, involves a systematic approach that ensures the reader actively interacts with the reading material, and thinks and reflects about what has been read. It involves trying to make sense of the material and constantly asking questions. When reading critically, it is important to make notes, as these will help promote thought and memory.

This template is a variation of the template on significant event analysis using similar (almost identical) headings. It is not necessarily clinically-based (unlike B14) and can be applied to any article.

B13 Critical reading

Title:
Author:
Journal:
Date read:

Why did you choose to read this article and what questions did you want answered?

Briefly summarise the article you have read: What was the article about?

Describe your feelings: How did the article make you feel?

Make a judgement: What were the positive aspects of this article, e.g. what did you find useful or interesting? What were the negative aspects of this article, e.g. what did you find unclear, not interesting or difficult?

Analyse: Did this article help you in your work? Were your questions answered?

Draw a conclusion: What can you conclude from reading this article? List the main learning points.

Make an action learning plan: Is there anything you need to address? Any learning needs identified or changes to the way you work?

B14 Critical reading: scientific/clinical articles

B14 is a template that is more specifically aimed at the critical reading of scientific/clinical articles. It has been adapted from *Critical Reading for the Reflective Practitioner.*[29] You are guided through a systematic approach with a number of prompts to help you reflect critically on any articles that you have read.

B14 Critical reading: scientific/clinical articles

Date read: Title: Author(s): Journal (ref):	
General aim • Why was the study done? • Why was it considered important?	
Specific objective • What was the specific question or questions being addressed by this particular study?	

The study setting • Where was the study done?	
The study population • To whom were the results of this study meant to apply (intended target population)? • What was the population first used in the study (the sampling population)? • What was the population that was finally studied (the study population)?	

The design

- What did the researchers do:

  Did they observe (observational study) or introduce a procedure or treatment (intervention study)?

  In what timeframe did they conduct the study: in current time (cross-sectional); looking back in time (retrospective); forward in time (prospective)?

  Was a comparison between two or more groups used (controlled) or no comparison made (uncontrolled)?

  Was the study group randomly selected for intervention (randomised) or not (non-randomised)?

The methods • What was or were: – the intervention (if appropriate)? – the baseline measurements? – the outcome measures (primary or secondary)?	
The results • Summarise those relevant to the study objective	
Authors' conclusions • Summarise the main points	

B15 Consultation analysis: video analysis

Learning about the consultation is best done in small groups. In the context of individuals showing videos to other members of the group, certain precautions need to be taken to ensure respect and honesty and ensure that the exercise is a learning one and not a frightening one.

It is therefore recommended that when viewing a video in a group, 'Pendleton's Rules' are observed.[30] These are:

1 The person showing the video clarifies any matters of fact about the patient or the surgery session.

2 The person showing the video then identifies what went well within the consultation, i.e. the strengths.

3 The group respond by adding their comments on what went well.

4 The person showing the video then focuses on what did not go so well or what could be improved upon.

5 The group then provides further comments on what did not go so well and what could be improved upon.

6 The person showing the video should be left with a statement of his/her strengths and what specific changes could lead to an improvement.

An alternative approach is to use the slightly modified ASDA Cambridge–Calgary approach to consultation analysis.[31, 32, 33]

- **Ask the group for help.** Choose a specific issue that has caused you concern and ask the group to help you with this problem. Try to be specific: 'My problem is . . .' or 'I would like help with . . .'
- **Specify the desired outcome.** Identify what you wish to learn or have achieved by the end of the presentation.
- **Describe accurately what occurs and the consequences.** View the tape and everyone should note what happened. Interpretation should be minimal but you should reflect on the consequences of the interventions.
- **Act out alternative suggestions.** The group should help you develop alternative

approaches. These should ideally be acted out in role play. Has your desired outcome been addressed? If yes, how? And if not, what would help you achieve your desired outcome?

You could present a video of your consultations to a group of your peers and use this guide for feedback and assessment.

B15 Consultation analysis: video analysis

The Calgary–Cambridge Observation Guide[32, 33]

Date: . . . .

Tasks	Achieved well	Areas for improvement
Initiating the session • Establishing initial rapport • Identifying the reason(s) for the consultation		
Gathering the information • Exploration of problems • Understanding the patient's perspective • Providing structure to the consultation		
Building the relationship • Developing rapport • Involving the patient		
Explanation and planning • Providing the correct amount and type of information • Aiding accurate recall and understanding		

• Achieving a shared understanding: incorporating the patient's perspective • Planning: shared decision making • Options in explanation and planning: – if discussing opinion and significance of problems – if negotiating mutual plan of action – if discussing investigations and procedures		
Closing the session		

Section C: Learning from our personal experiences and life events

A great deal can be learnt from experiences of life outside your professional sphere. You reflect and use this learning and this helps to shape how you behave as a human being and as a health professional. You learn from your relationships with other people, from your partners, from your parents, from being a parent and from your children. You may have experienced major life events such as moving house, changing jobs, getting married, ending a relationship, births and deaths. You will have had joyous moments and sad and difficult times. You are no different to the patients that consult you. You share with them the same experiences and whilst your own experiences are poignant and personal, how you interpret and make sense of them has particular relevance to your work.

Recording these events and how you reacted to and reflected upon them can be helpful in making sense of patients' sufferings. In this section you could include anything of a personal nature (becoming or being a parent, being a carer, experiencing bereavement) if you feel it has helped you become who you are. It need not necessarily be in a written form. You may for example wish to include a photograph or an object, which may say it all for you.

Because of their personal nature, you may regard these reflections as confidential and of no concern to other people. This should not necessarily prevent you from introducing them into your portfolio. (If you wish, you can always remove them if other people are to look at your portfolio.)

You also learn a great deal from outside the sphere of medicine and health. This also contributes to how you behave and relate to other people. You can obtain a great deal of insight into patients, their illnesses and the way that you interact and communicate with them, from reading general fiction and non-fiction (prose, poetry and drama). Reading can help develop a broader perspective of the world and increase your understanding of life. It can introduce alternative ways of seeing, feeling and understanding.

The Archers has been on the radio for 50 years. When it first came on the air, it had a specific objective of educating the post-war population about farming methods. But over the years, the programme has broadened and has dealt with many contemporary social issues. Most recently, Ruth Archer, mother of two young children, has developed breast cancer. The programme deals with the issues around diagnosis, dealing with uncertainty, breaking bad news, mastectomy and so on. As a health professional, you see your patients when they present to you in illness. You may hear from them about the effects of their illness on themselves, their family and their friends, but you are not a direct witness to these effects. A programme such as *The Archers*, dealing with these issues, offers a rare opportunity to understand and empathise with patients.

Even before Ruth Archer's breast cancer, a doctor wrote in the *BMJ* of how he had learnt about a character's illness and treatment from listening to *The Archers*.[34] He wondered if this learning could earn him points for his continuing medical education (or entertainment). And why not?

In this section, you could include any examples you wish to contribute from literature (fiction, non-fiction, biography), drama or poetry. You may also wish to include learning from art, films, television, radio or the theatre.

Section D: Addressing clinical governance

Quality assurance

Provide a summary of how you have addressed this area and include examples/evidence of any of the following in your portfolio:

- examples of evidence-based practice, e.g. critical reading of evidence-based literature, use of evidence-based websites, application of evidence-based guidelines
- opportunities to discuss and respond to national guidelines (NICE, NSFs), e.g. practice meetings, incorporation of guidelines
- opportunities to discuss and respond to local guidelines, e.g. practice meetings, incorporation of guidelines
- development of in-house standards, protocols or guidelines, e.g. include examples
- training programmes relevant to quality assurance, e.g. in-house or external
- evidence of review of quality assurance
- examples of critical reading
- continuing education and training programmes
- review of complaints, e.g. learning from complaints/mistakes
- patient views and involving patients, e.g. suggestions box, patients' association.

Clinical audit

In this section provide examples of audits that you have carried out. If you complete A15 and include this in your portfolio, it will address all the relevant and important issues.

Clinical effectiveness

Provide a summary of how you have addressed this area and include examples/ evidence of any of the following in your portfolio:

- examples of evidence-based practice, e.g. critical reading of evidence-based literature, use of evidence-based websites, application of evidence-based guidelines
- opportunities to discuss and respond to national guidelines (NICE, NSFs), e.g. practice meetings, incorporation of guidelines
- opportunities to discuss and respond to local guidelines
- development of in-house standards, protocols or guidelines
- training programmes relevant to clinical effectiveness
- evidence of review of clinical effectiveness
- examples of critical reading.

Clinical risk management

Provide a summary of how you have addressed this area and include examples/ evidence of any of the following in your portfolio:

- access issues such as provision for the disabled, telephone access, appointment availability, dealing with emergencies
- health and safety policies such as infection control, clinical waste management, needle stick injury, equipment maintenance, fire procedures, dealing with difficult/aggressive patients
- clinical issues such as safe prescribing – acute and repeat prescriptions, dealing with referrals, emergency drug and resuscitation equipment maintenance
- medical records, use of computers, maintaining confidentiality
- significant event analysis
- training in CPR/anaphylaxis
- patient complaint procedures
- patient liaison groups.

Staff and organisational development

Provide a summary of how you have addressed this area and include examples/ evidence of any of the following in your portfolio:

- examples of job descriptions/contracts
- examples of training and continuing education
- personal or practice development plans
- portfolios
- policies of recruitment
- appraisal or peer review systems
- teambuilding exercises
- primary healthcare team meetings.

Part Four

Appendices

Appendix 1
Teacher portfolios

Accountability does not only apply to clinical areas within the NHS. Teachers are not exempt. They need to expose themselves to scrutiny both as health professionals and as teachers. They will be accountable to their accrediting bodies and through them to the public, who have a right to know that high quality standards are being applied to the training of PHCT staff.

In primary care the teaching of medicine occurs at undergraduate and postgraduate levels. Systems for the certification and re-certification of postgraduate GP teachers have been in existence for a number of years. As increasing amounts of the undergraduate curriculum are being taught in primary care, there is a need to increase the numbers of undergraduate GP teachers. The training, certification and re-certification of undergraduate GP teachers is, in many cases, not fully developed and in some parts of the country has yet to be established. In the primary healthcare setting, teaching of other health professionals is not as structured or formalised. In both undergraduate and postgraduate teaching, it is not only the teacher who is accredited, but also the practice (PHCT) which has a pivotal role in the delivery of the teaching. Therefore, all members of a PHCT in an accredited teaching practice should be involved in teaching.

If teachers are to successfully promote the concepts of adult learning, which encourages autonomy and self-direction, they need to embrace these theories themselves. They should be involved in critical reflection, designing their own learning contracts or education plans and should also engage in self-appraisal of their teaching skills. A teacher portfolio is more than a 'mere listing of activities as in a curriculum vitae; it is a compilation of intentions, strategic actions and reflections'.[35] It should provide evidence of quality in a teacher through the demonstration of:

- effective communication skills
- enthusiasm and motivation
- good knowledge of the subject

- planning and delivery of a curriculum
- range of appropriate teaching methods and skills
- awareness of pastoral needs of their learners
- ability to provide a range of meaningful assessment tools and provide effective feedback
- involvement in critical reflection and self-appraisal
- commitment to lifelong learning and developing education plans.

A suggested proforma for a teacher portfolio is included which may be modified for individual use.

Suggested proforma for a teacher portfolio

1   Introduction

1.1 CV to include past teaching and research experience.
1.2 Current clinical practices/service development.

2 Current teaching practice

2.1 Undergraduate.
2.2 Postgraduate.
2.3 Administrative role.
2.4 Outside teaching.
2.5 Support provided for others (mentorship/supervision).
2.6 Other.

3 Evaluation of teaching – quantitative/qualitative

3.1 Student evaluation of teaching.
3.2 Course evaluation.
3.3 Peer appraisal.
3.4 Student achievement.
3.5 Self-assessment.
3.6 Assessment work.

4 Reflective practice

4.1 Significant event audit.
4.2 Critical reading.
4.3 Courses/workshops attended.
4.4 Responsiveness to self/peer assessment.
4.5 Teaching improvements and innovations.
4.6 Evaluation of personal development plan.

5 Research

5.1 Education.
5.2 Clinical.
5.3 Grants.
5.4 Other.

6 Personal development plan

6.1 What do I need to learn?
6.2 What are the outcomes or benefits?
6.3 How will I do it? What resources are needed?
6.4 How will I show what I have learnt? What will the outcome look like?
6.5 How will I and my teaching practice benefit?

Appendix 2
Revalidation for doctors

The General Medical Council (GMC) has published its proposals for the revalidation of doctors.[3] Doctors will be required to provide evidence of their continuing fitness to practice in the form of a folder (i.e. a portfolio).* The method of revalidation (i.e. a portfolio) is unlikely to change although the contents of the portfolio, suggested by the GMC, may alter following consultation. It is intended that the portfolio will be divided into five sections and contain information concerning personal and performance issues. The five sections are listed below together with suggestions as to how the toolbox *can* help provide the evidence.

Personal details

This concerns your personal details, qualifications, date of last revalidation and registration details (including breaks, conditions imposed or suspensions).

The personal profile in Part 2 addresses this section.

What the doctor does

This section requests information regarding your current practice, any other appointments held and time spent on clinical and non-clinical work.

The personal and practice profile in Part 2 addresses this section.

Information about performance

Here information is required regarding good clinical care, keeping up to date, working with colleagues, teaching and training, relationships with patients, probity and health.

Nearly all of the templates address this section, for example clinical care and keeping up to date is covered by most. See also teaching and training (Appendix 1) and the specific templates for relationships with patients and probity (A13, A14, B8, B9), critical incidents (A4) and complaints (A5).

How the doctor can improve

This is a request for information on how you can improve upon performance through the conditions in which you work and through identifying and acting upon any training and development needs. It asks you to develop an action plan (with a timeframe).

A personal and a practice education plan (A2, A10, B2).

Statement signed

Finally, you and your appraiser are requested to sign a statement confirming that the information in the portfolio has been reviewed.

* There may be circumstances under which a doctor would present evidence of fitness to practice based on an objective assessment of ability rather than a folder of evidence.

Appendix 3
Useful names, addresses and websites

Audit Commission
1 Vincent Square
London SW1 2PN
Tel: 020 7828 1212
Fax: 020 7976 6187
Website: http://www.auditcommission.gov.uk

Bandolier
Pain Relief Unit
The Churchill Hospital
Headington
Oxford OX3 7LJ
Tel: 01865 226 132
Fax: 01865 226 978
Website: http://www.jr2.ox.ac.uk/bandolier

British Medical Association
(*British Medical Journal*)
BMA House
Tavistock Square
London WC1H 9JP
Tel: 020 7387 4499
Fax: 020 7383 6406
Website: http://bma.org.uk
          (http://www.bmj.com)

Centre for Evidence-Based Medicine
Radcliffe Hospital
Headley Way
Headington
Oxford OX3 9DU
Tel: 01865 741 166
Fax: 01865 741 408
Website: http://cebm.jr2.ox.ac.uk/

Centre for Evidence-Based Nursing
The Department of Health Studies
Innovation Centre
York Science Park
University Road
York YO10 5DG
Tel: 01904 435 222
Fax: 01904 435 225
Website: http://www.york.ac.uk/depts/hstd/centres/evidence/ev-intro.htm

Centre for Innovation in Primary Care
First Floor
Walsh Court
Sheffield S1 2FY
Tel: 0114 220 2000
Fax: 0114 220 2001
Website: http://www.innovate.org.uk

Clinical Governance Research and Development Unit
See National Clinical Audit Centre

Clinical Practice Evaluation Programme (CPEP)
School of Health and Related Research
University of Sheffield
Regent Court
Sheffield S1 4DA
Tel: 0114 222 0812
Fax: 0114 222 0791
Website: http://www.shef.ac.uk/~schar/publich/cpep

Community Practitioners and Health Visitors Association
36 Eccleston Square
London SW1 1PF
Tel: 020 7939 7000
Fax: 020 7403 2976
Website: http://www.msfcphva.org

Contacts, Help, Advice and Information Network (CHAIN)
c/o Research and Development
London Regional Office
40 Eastbourne Terrace
London WC2 3QR
Tel: 020 7725 5535
Fax: 020 7725 5655
Website: http://www.nthames-health.tpmde.ac.uk/chain/introduction.htm

Cochrane Library
Summertown Pavilion
Middle Way
Oxford OX2 7LG
Tel: 01865 523 902
Fax: 01865 516 918
Website: http://www.update-software.com/ccweb/default.html

Data Protection Register
Springfield House
Water Lane
Wilmslow
Cheshire SK9 5AX
Tel: 01625 545 745
Fax: 01625 545 510
Website: http://www.dataprotection.co.uk

Database of Abstracts of Reviews of Effectiveness (DARE)
See NHS Centre for Reviews and Dissemination

Department of Health
PO Box 777
London SE1 6XH
Tel: 0800 555 777
Fax: 01623 724 524
Website: http://www.doh.gov.uk

Doctors desk
Tel: 020 8725 5661
Fax: 020 8767 7697
Website: http://www.drsdesk.sghms.ac.uk

Doctors.net.uk
Freepost (SCE6579)
Abingdon
Oxon OX14 4YG
Tel: 01235 828 400
Fax: 01235 862 791
Website: http://www.doctors.net.uk

General Medical Council
178 Great Portland Street
London W1N 6JE
Tel: 020 7580 7642
Fax: 020 7915 3641
Website: http://www.gmc-uk.org

Institute of Healthcare Management
7–10 Chandos Street
London W1M 9DE
Tel: 020 7460 7654
Fax: 020 7460 7655
Website: http://www.ihm.org.uk

King's Fund
11–13 Cavendish Square
London W1M 0AN
Tel: 020 7307 2400
Fax: 020 7307 2801
Website: http://www.kingsfund.org.uk

Medical Defence Union
230 Blackfriars Road
London SE1 8PG
Tel: 020 7202 1500
Fax: 020 7202 1666
Website: http://www.the-mdu.com

Medical Protection Society
33 Cavendish Square
London W1M 0PS
Tel: 020 7399 1300
Fax: 020 7399 1301
Website: http://www.mps.org.uk

Medical Research Council
20 Park Crescent
London W1N 4AL
Tel: 020 7636 5422
Fax: 020 7436 6179
Website: http://www.mrc.ac.uk

National Association of Patient Participation
PO Box 999
Nuneaton
Warks CV11 5ZD
Tel: 0151 630 5786
Fax: 0151 630 5786
Website: http://www.napp.org.uk

NHS Centre for Reviews and Dissemination (CRD)
University of York Information Service
Heslington
York YO1 5DD
Tel: 01904 434 555
Fax: 01904 433 661
Website: http://www.york.ac.uk/inst/crd/

NHS Executive
Department of Health
Quarry House
Quarry Hill
Leeds LS2 7UE
Tel: 0113 254 5610
Website: http://www.doh.gov.uk/pricare

National Clinical Audit Centre
Department of General Practice and Primary Health Care
University of Leicester
Leicester General Hospital
Leicester LE5 4PW
Tel: 0116 258 4873
Fax: 0116 258 4982
Website: http://www.le.ac.uk/cgrdu

National Counselling Service for Sick Doctors
First Assist
Wheatfield Way
Hinkley
Leicestershire LE10 1YG
Tel: 08702 410 535
Fax: 01455 254 027

National Institute for Clinical Excellence
90 Long Acre
Covent Garden
London WC2E 9RF
Tel: 020 7383 6451
Fax: 020 7849 3127
Website: http://www.nice.org.uk

National Primary Care Research and Development Centre (NPCRDC)
The University of Manchester
Williamson Building
Oxford Road
Manchester M13 9PL
Tel: 0161 275 7601
Fax: 0161 275 7600
Website: http://www.npcrdc.man.ac.uk

Prescription Pricing Authority
Scottish Life House
Archbold Terrace
Jesmond
Newcastle upon Tyne NE2 1DB
Tel: 0191 203 5000
Fax: 0191 203 5001
Website: http://www.ppa.org.uk

Royal College of General Practitioners
14 Princes Gate
Hyde Park
London SW7 1PU
Tel: 020 7581 3232
Fax: 020 7225 3047
Website: http://www.rcgp.org.uk

Royal College of Midwives
15 Mansfield Street
London W1M 0BE
Tel: 020 7312 3535
Fax: 020 7312 3536
Website: http://www.rcm.org.uk

Royal College of Nursing
20 Cavendish Square
London W1M 0AB
Tel: 020 7409 3333
Fax: 020 7647 3435
Website: http://www.rcn.org.uk

UKCC
23 Portland Place
London W1N 4JT
Tel: 020 7637 7181
Fax: 020 7436 2924
Website: http://www.ukcc.org.uk

References

1 Department of Health (1998) *A Review of Continuing Professional Development in General Practice.* A report by the Chief Medical Officer. Department of Health, London.

2 Secretary of State for Health (1998) *A First Class Service: quality in the new NHS.* Department of Health, London.

3 General Medical Council (2000) *Revalidation for Doctors: ensuring standards, securing the future.* General Medical Council, London.

4 Knowles M (1990) *The Adult Learner: a neglected species.* Gulf Publishing, Houston.

5 Boud D, Keogh R and Walker D (1985) *Reflection: turning experience into learning.* Kogan Page, London.

6 McGill I and Beaty L (1995) *Action Learning.* Kogan Page, London.

7 Kolb DA (1985) *Experiential Learning: experience as the source of learning.* Prentice-Hall, London.

8 Gibbs G (1990) *Learning by Doing: a guide to teaching and learning methods.* FEU, London.

9 Langsdorf L (1988) Ethical and logical analysis as human science. *Human Studies.* 11: 45.

10 Brookfield SD (1987) *Developing Critical Thinkers: challenging adults to explore alternative ways of thinking and acting.* Jossey Bass, San Francisco.

11 Royal College of General Practitioners (1993) *Portfolio-based learning in general practice.* Occasional Paper No. 63. RCGP, London.

12 Pietroni RG and Millard L (1996) Portfolio-based learning. In: J Hasler and D Pendleton (eds) *Professional Development in General Practice.* Oxford University Press, Oxford.

13 Luft J (1984) *Group Processes: an introduction to group dynamics.* Mayfield, California.

14 Freeman R (1998) *Mentoring in General Practice.* Butterworth Heinemann, Oxford.

15 Rogers C (1983) *Freedom to Learn for the Eighties.* Charles E Merrill, Ohio.

16 Maynard T and Furlong J (1995) Learning to teach and models of mentoring.

In: T Kerry and A Shelton Mayes (eds) *Issues in Mentoring*. Routledge, London.

17 Pietroni RG and Palmer A (1995) Portfolio based learning and the role of mentors. *Postgraduate Education for General Practice*. **6**: 111–14.

18 Davies HTO and Nutley SM (2000) Developing learning organisations in the new NHS. *BMJ*. **320**: 998–1001.

19 Davies C (2000) Getting health professionals to work together. *BMJ*. **320**: 1021–22.

20 Leathard A (ed) (1994) *Going Inter-Professional: working together for health and welfare*. Routledge, London.

21 Pedler M, Burgoyne J and Boydell T (1996) *The Learning Company*. McGraw-Hill, New York.

22 Senge PM (1994) *The Fifth Discipline: the art and practice of the learning organisation currency*. Doubleday, New York.

23 Davies HTO and Nutley SM (2000) Organisational culture and quality of health care. *Quality in Health Care*. **9**: 111–19.

24 Hayes ME (1987) *Make Every Minute Count: how to manage your time effectively*. Kogan Page, London.

25 Pringle M, Bradley C, Carmichael C *et al*. (1995) *Significant Event Auditing*. Occasional Paper No. 70. RCGP, London.

26 Tripp D (1993) *Critical Incidents in Teaching: developing professional judgement*. Routledge, London.

27 Howie JGR, Heaney DJ, Maxwell M and Walker JJ (1998) A comparison of the Patient Enablement Instrument (PEI) against two established satisfaction scales as an outcome measure of primary care consultations. *Family Practice*. **15**: 165–71.

28 Greco M, Cavanagh M, Bownlea A and McGovern J (1999) The Doctor's Interpersonal Skills Questionnaire (DISQ): a validated instrument for use in GP training. *Education for General Practice*. **10**: 256–64.

29 Clarke R and Croft P (1998) *Critical Reading for the Reflective Practitioner*. Butterworth Heinemann, Oxford.

30 Pendleton D, Schofield T, Tate P and Havelock P (1984) *The Consultation: an approach to learning and teaching*. Oxford University Press, Oxford.

31 Kurtz SM and Silverman JD (1996) Cambridge Calgary approach to consultation analysis. *Education for General Practice*. **7**: 288–99.

32 Kurtz SM, Silverman JD and Draper J (1998) *Teaching and Learning Communication Skills in Medicine.* Radcliffe Medical Press, Oxford.

33 Silverman JD, Kurtz SM and Draper J (1998) *Skills for Communicating with Patients.* Radcliffe Medical Press, Oxford.

34 Bolton J (2000) How about earning points for continuing medical entertainment? *BMJ.* **320**: 1408.

35 Nightingale P and O'Neil M (1994) *Achieving Quality Learning in Higher Education.* Kogan Page, London.

Index

accountability 33
  clinical governance 18
  NHS 43
  for quality of service 37
  teachers 175
action learning 7–8
action plans *see* personal education
      (development or action) plans
acute care audits *88–9*
addresses 181–8
administrative environment 50
adult learning 7–13
appraisals 127–8
  from others *133–4*
  self-appraisals *see* self-appraisals
  skills related *135–42*
apprenticeship model, mentoring 31
articles, critical reading 156, *157–60*
audits
  clinical 47–8, 168
  learning from 87
    acute care *88–9*
    chronic care *88–9*
    practice management *90–1*
    screening and prevention *90–1*

brainstorming 27

Calgary–Cambridge Observation Guide *163–4*
CHI (Commission for Health Improvement)
      45
chronic care audits *88–9*
clinical articles, critical reading 156, *157–60*
clinical audits 47–8, 168

clinical effectiveness 48–9, 169
clinical governance 1, 33
  applying 18–19
  clinical audit 47–8, 168
  clinical effectiveness 48–9, 169
  clinical risk management 49, 170
  continuing education links 44
  definition 43
  delivery 44–5
  development links 44
  evidence, portfolios as 44
  organisational development 50–1, 171
  quality 45–6
  quality assurance 46–7, 167
  staff development 50–1, 171
  standards 46–7
  structures for delivery 44–5
  training links 44
clinical risk management 49, 170
clinical topics, identifying individual strengths
      92–3, *94–5*
collaborative working 34
colleagues, learning from 17–18, 109–64
Commission for Health Improvement (CHI) 45
competency model, mentoring 31
complaints, learning from 83, *84*
confidentiality of portfolio entries 38, 165
consultation analysis
  patient assessment 102, *103–4*
  self-assessment 98, *99–101*
  video analysis 161–2, *163–4*
contents of portfolios 15–16
continuing development 22

continuing education 37
   clinical governance links 44
   evidence, portfolios as 44
continuing professional development (CPD) 1
courses, learning from 118, *119–21*
critical reading 152, *153–5*
   scientific/clinical articles 156, *157–60*
critical reflection 9–11
cultural transformation 36
culture, organisational 33–4

dating entries in portfolios 38
development
   clinical governance links 44
   continuing 1, 22
   organisational 50–1, 171
   plans *see* personal education (development
      or action) plans; practice education (or
      development) plans
   portfolios as logs of 20
   professional 37
   staff 50–1, 171
   doctors' interpersonal skills questionnaires
      (DISQ) 102, *104*
   doctors' revalidation *see* revalidation for
      doctors

education
   in-house events 124, *125–6*
   see also continuing education; personal
      education (development or action)
      plans; practice education (or
      development) plans; training
effectiveness, clinical 48–9, 169
errors *see* mistakes
evaluation of learning 26
evidence, portfolios as 44
evidence of learning achievements 25
external guidelines 146, *147–8*
externally based standards 47

feelings about learning experiences 10

governance *see* clinical governance
guidelines
   development of 143, *144–5*
   external, learning from 146, *147–8*

health improvement programmes (HImP) 47
helpers 13
   roles 29–31
HImP (health improvement programmes) 47

in-house education events 124, *125–6*
individual strengths and weaknesses *see*
      strengths; weaknesses
inter-professional learning 122, *123*
internally based standards 46
interpersonal skills questionnaires, doctors'
      (DISQ) 102, *104*
investment in learning 35

Johari window 22–4

learning
   on action 7–8
   contracts *see* personal education
      (development or action) plans
   evaluation of 26
   evidence of achievements 25
   feelings about experiences 10
   framework for recording 16
   investment in 35
   objectives 25
   needs
      identification 21–4, 26
      patient interaction logs 78, *79*
   portfolio-based 12–13
   re-evaluating experiences 10–11
   reflection 7–8
   remembering and recollecting experiences
      9–10
   resources, needs 25
   self-assessment of needs 21–4

sources
    colleagues 17–18, 109–64
    negatives 83, *84–5*
    patients 8, 17, 71–108
    personal life experiences 12, 18, 165–6
    work 8–9
learning environment 50–1
learning organisations 34–6
lectures 8
    learning from 118, *119–21*
life experiences, learning from 12, 18, 165–6
listening 30–1
locally based standards 47

management of risk *see* risk management
management of time 11, 37–8, 39
meetings, learning from 118, *119–21*
mentoring 30–1
    see also helpers
mistakes
    learning from 83, *85*
    prevention 49
    reflection on 9

names, addresses and websites 181–8
National Health Service (NHS)
    accountability 43
National Institute for Clinical Excellence
        (NICE) 45
National Service Frameworks (NSFs) 45, 146
near misses, learning from 83, *85*
negative synergy 34
negatives, learning from 83, *84–5*
NHS *see* National Health Service
NICE (National Institute for Clinical
        Excellence) 45
non-clinical topics, identifying individual
        strengths 72–3, *74–5*
NSFs (National Service Frameworks) 45, 146

objectives, learning 25

organisational culture 33–4
organisational development 50–1, 171
outside events, learning from 118, *119–21*

PACT (prescribing analysis and cost) data
        105, *106–8*
patient assessment consultation analysis 102,
        103–4
patient enablement instrument (PEI) 102, *103*
patient interaction logs 78, *79*
patients, learning from 8, 17, 71–108
PEI (patient enablement instrument) 102, *103*
Pendleton's Rules 161
personal education (development or action)
        plans 24–7, 72–3, *76–7*, 93, *96–7*
personal life experiences, learning from 12, 18,
        165–6
personal profiles *55–9*
PGEA (postgraduate education allowance)
        11–12
PHCT *see* primary healthcare teams
physical environment 50
physical form of portfolios 40
planning
    time management 11
    see also personal education (development or
        action) plans; practice education (or
        development) plans
portfolio-based learning 12–13
portfolios
    confidentiality 38, 165
    contents 15–16
    dating entries 38
    development, logs of 20
    as evidence for clinical governance,
        revalidation and continuing education
        44
    nature 11
    physical form 40
    teachers 175–7
    tips on keeping 40–1

positive synergy 34
positives, learning from 86
postgraduate education allowance (PGEA) 11–12
PPA (Prescription Pricing Authority) 105
practice education (or development) plans 26–7, 111, 113, *116–17*
practice management audits *90–1*
practice profiles *61–5*
practices
  sharing education and continuing development 124, *125–6*
  strengths and weaknesses 110, 112–13, *114–15*
prescribing analysis and cost (PACT) data 105, *106–8*
prescribing units (PU) 105
Prescription Pricing Authority (PPA) 105
prevention audits *90–1*
primary healthcare teams (PHCT)
  see also practice education (or development) plans
  learning needs 26–7
  learning organisations 33–6
  sharing experiences and learning 19
prioritising 11
professional development 37
profiles
  personal *55–9*
  practice *61–5*
protocols, development of 143, *144–5*
PU (prescribing units) 105

quality assurance
  clinical governance 46–7, 167
quality of care 37, 43, 44, 45–6

re-evaluating learning experiences 10–11
reading *see* critical reading
reciprocal mentoring 31
recollecting learning experiences 9–10

reflection
  critical 9–11
  on learning 7–8
  on mistakes 9
  time for 11
reflective practitioner model, mentoring 31
regionally based standards 47
remembering learning experiences 9–10
resources, needs 25
revalidation for doctors 1
  portfolios as evidence 44, 179–80
reviewing learning plans 25
risk management 49, 170
  learning from 149, *150–1*

scientific articles, critical reading 156, *157–60*
Scottish Health Technologies Assessment Centre (SHTAC) 45
screening audits *90–1*
self-appraisals *129–32*
  of strengths and weaknesses 72–3, *74–5*, 92–3, *94–5*
self-assessment
  consultation analysis 98, *99–101*
  of learning needs 21–4
SHTAC (Scottish Health Technologies Assessment Centre) 45
significant event analysis 80, *81–2*
'sitting with Nellie' 31
skills
  appraisals *135–42*
  doctors' interpersonal skills questionnaires (DISQ) 102, *104*
staff development 50–1, 171
standards, clinical governance 46–7
strengths 26–7
  individual, identifying
    clinical topics 92–3, *94–5*
    non-clinical topics 72–3, *74–5*
  learning from 86
  practice, identifying 110, 112–13, *114–15*

structures for delivery of clinical governance
    44–5
SWOT analyses 26–7, 72, 92, 110
synergy, positive and negative 34

teacher portfolios 175–7
teaching practices 175
teamwork 19, 34
    see also primary healthcare teams
templates
    learning from colleagues 109–64
    learning from patients 71–108
    use 16, 19, 69–70
time
    for reflection 11
    management 11, 37–8, 39
training
    see also personal education (development or

action) plans; practice education (or
    development) plans
clinical governance links 44
clinical risk management 49
undergraduate GP teachers 175

useful names, addresses and websites 181–8

video analysis 161–2, *163–4*

weaknesses 26–7
    individual, identifying
        clinical topics 92–3, *94–5*
        non-clinical topics 72–3, *74–5*
    practice, identifying 110, 112–13, *114–15*
website addresses 181–8
work, as source of learning 87–104